ALSO BY DR. PHIL McGRAW

WE'VE GOT ISSUES

How You Can Stand Strong for
America's Soul and Sanity

Phillip C. McGraw, Ph.D.

THRESHOLD EDITIONS

New York   London   Toronto   Sydney   New Delhi

Threshold Editions
An Imprint of Simon & Schuster, LLC
1230 Avenue of the Americas
New York, NY 10020

Copyright © 2024 by Phillip C. McGraw

First Threshold Editions hardcover edition February 2024

THRESHOLD EDITIONS and colophon are trademarks of Simon & Schuster, LLC

Simon & Schuster: Celebrating 100 Years of Publishing in 2024

An index for this title can be found at simonandschuster.com and drphil.com

For information about special discounts for bulk purchases, please contact Simon & Schuster Special Sales at 1-866-506-1949 or business@simonandschuster.com.

The Simon & Schuster Speakers Bureau can bring authors to your live event. For more information or to book an event, contact the Simon & Schuster Speakers Bureau at 1-866-248-3049 or visit our website at www.simonspeakers.com.

Manufactured in the United States of America

10 9 8 7 6 5 4 3 2 1

Library of Congress Cataloging-in-Publication Data has been applied for.

ISBN 978-1-6680-6170-1
ISBN 978-1-6680-6172-5 (ebook)

I dedicate this book to my wife and entire family who always support me in all that I do even though that sometimes brings controversy to our doorsteps—especially for letting all sides have an opportunity to express their views in open debate;

And to

All of those committed Americans who love their family and their country despite being judged for how they do it.

Contents

A Letter from Dr. Phil

Dear Reader,

Before I start this book in earnest, permit me a personal note. You may be familiar with me or not. For the purposes of this book, it doesn't matter.

I've been on television for years, sometimes more than fifty hours a week, mostly talking to real people looking for real solutions to real problems.

I haven't always gotten it perfectly right, but I have always shared the truth, whether it was what people wanted to hear or not. I take what I do *very* seriously and have spent twenty-five years listening intently to our guests and millions of viewers and studying the important psychosocial issues and trends in American society. Those issues and trends have changed dramatically over the last several years, first somewhat gradually, now anything but. Many of the trends I address in this book are not a result of society's natural evolution, but have been in my opinion unquestionably designed to undermine our society in general and the family unit in particular. There can be no other explanation. I intend to prove that to you based on hard evidence. I expect much of what I share will leave you shocked and dismayed. In the end I hope your attitude will be "Sorry to hear it but very glad to know it." Because "knowing it" means you can start changing things for you and your family. You have one life to live; there's no dress rehearsal. I want to help you make this one count.

Activists, with what many in the political arena call "woke" agendas, are on the attack. They and their acolytes seem to have entered our lives and our national conversation in such an aggressive way that loud gets confused with laudable and verbosity is mistaken for validity. These fringe factions are pushing toxic ideologies in areas critical to both your personal life and our national life in every way they can.

Their goal is to erase boundary lines so you can then be called on and expected to *join with them*. Just look at education, from kindergarten all the way through our universities. I believe we actually have activists training our teachers especially on issues involving gender and race, and asking you to let them coparent your own child on important social and developmental issues!

I believe these activists are preying on our children at a time when they are at their most vulnerable, while their brains are still developing. No wonder our children are suffering record-high levels of depression, anxiety, and loneliness.

If we remain silent—or even quietly submissive—we sacrifice not only our children's future but also the future of our country.

Chapter by chapter, I will show you the results of a survey conducted specifically for this book that reveal that too many of us may be aware of but yet reluctant to speak up about what's happening all around us for fear of being targeted, labeled as "phobic," or unenlightened—and being "cancelled."

Disruptive activists are even invading the practice of medicine, usurping science by putting social pressure on medical decisions for such things as "gender-affirming care" for children. So it is not just an attack on individual thought and values: institutional standards, values, practices, and canons of ethics are being targeted as well.

It doesn't stop there.

Since our founding, this country has embraced cultural philosophies that have set us apart from so many other countries and cultures. At its core, America is built on the idea of meritocracy, founded on the principles of rewarding hard work and talent. Those who added value would reap rewards. Those who didn't, wouldn't. Not so much anymore.

Historically, those who broke the law paid a price. We always recognized there would be consequences for criminals. Not so much anymore.

Now we barely arrest the bad actors. These days, prosecutors and judges seem to think it more "enlightened" to focus on the ideology that the "system" failed the *criminal* as much as or more than the victim, downplaying or dispensing with personal accountability. I'm sure society does play a role in a criminal's poor choices, but no theory should outweigh personal responsibility. You hear the activists argue for the release of these criminals onto an unsuspecting and innocent society, even those with a history of violent, unprovoked assaults. What you don't hear or see is those same people showing up at the jail when these criminals are released saying, "Hey, come over to my house and hang out with me and my children."

We have always respected facts and science and embraced the truth. We believed those things that could be proven absent bias. Not so much anymore.

Now, if some group doesn't like the truth, they just pretend it isn't so and come up with a new set of words to describe what they wish was reality.

We are allowing loud people (that is, "activists") who in many instances I don't believe really even speak for those they purport to represent to change some core definitions of our culture, demagnetize our moral compass, and undercut the very cornerstones of our society and success.

All of them pursue a strategy that (and this is not a complete list) has at least three things in common:

➤ Make you feel guilty,

➤ Undermine the strength of your family, and

➤ Create new victim classes, all of whom want special attention and treatment.

As a father, grandfather, and husband of forty-seven years and counting—and a proud American—I am sensitive to what is happening. You might be surprised how many life experiences you and I have in common. I wasn't born "Dr. Phil." My boys always joke that I have "more degrees than a thermometer." But I can honestly say that a *lot* of what I know was not learned on the college campus, but from growing up in a dysfunctional family marred by alcoholism, chaos, and instability—at times so unstable I had no roof over my head at all. In retrospect I wonder if some of those times on my own weren't some of the most peaceful.

Looking back, I don't really regret those experiences all that much. I am glad our two boys didn't grow up the way I did, but for some reason it all seems to have worked for me. I believe everything I have ever done or experienced has prepared me for what I am now doing.

Some facts of life you learn only through experience and some lessons you can only teach yourself. When you grow up poor and have only yourself to rely on, you quickly learn to deal with reality. There is no room or time for fiction or fantasy. You measure things based on results. You can't pay your bills or buy food with what you meant to accomplish. You learn that what counts is what you actually got done. Hunger is a really good motivator!

My journey instilled in me several core beliefs:

- This is a great country where hard work really can pay off.

- Victimhood is a wasted mindset. Nobody really cares about your whining regardless of what they say to your face.

- *Misery is not a strategy.*

- An attitude of entitlement, a desire for a free ride will ruin your future and keep you from ever getting on your own two feet and marching forward on a true path to success.

- If you listen to nonsense and substitute other people's thinking for your own, you sacrifice self-determination and more often than not will be used and abused.

These beliefs are time-tested, and they are neither pessimistic nor optimistic; they are realistic. Yet I am still watching people stagnated, listening to nonsense, hoping for that free ride, expecting equality of outcome independent of their input. Yeah, well, good luck with that.

I hear politicians on both sides of the aisle telling us all, "This xyz program of *free services*—costing double-digit billions—won't cost you taxpayers one penny!" Every time I hear that kind of nonsense, I swear I want to grab a mirror and see if someone wrote "STUPID" on my forehead! I can't tell you how many times during the week I hear or read something and think, "Whoa! Time out! Grab the mirror!"

And I wonder if those advocating or promoting these programs actually *want* to foster dependency.

I believe if we don't stop this ideological invasion and stop it right now, we will collectively become a very different and weakened culture. I am not one to yell "Fire!" in a crowded theater. I am not one to overreact and cause panic. But if you are sensing urgency in my words, you are reading me right. I think "we," the vast majority of Americans—the mothers and fathers, grandmothers and grand-fathers, the folks who get up every day and go to work and pay our fair share and take pride in family, tradition, and country (including me)—are about ten years behind the curve and have allowed these toxic activists, however you choose to label them, to get a foothold in too many critical areas. We have to react now.

We have to wake up and stop giving in to the nonsense. So many of these "ideas" are simply made up; ideas that are miles away from reality and common sense—and yet those espousing them are demanding (and sometimes even attaining) acceptance. We cannot allow this to continue.

I refer to it as the "Tyranny of the Fringe." I believe we are in a full-blown culture war, and nobody has the luxury of being a non-combatant.

Over half of the people in a recent poll admitted they were too intimidated to even ask questions because that can get you "can-celled." And God forbid you go so far as to speak out against any of the ideologies being crammed down your throats.

We are going to talk about the reality involved in raising a family in today's America. The fears associated with simply speaking up, and the intimidation felt regarding all the words we supposedly can't use because even if uttered in benign ignorance they can result in being "cancelled" and labeled a "hater."

Please understand, I'm not content to just complain and find fault. It's like Sam Rayburn, the long-serving Speaker of the House and proud Texan, used to say: "Any jackass can kick down a barn, but it takes a carpenter to build one." I want to be a carpenter!

And I want you to be one too.

To help you do that at certain points in the book, I'm going to ask you to write things down: your values, thoughts, beliefs.

I'm also going to be asking you to take a few surveys, and show you as we go along how to profile yourself in comparison to thousands of others regarding how you think and feel in your approach to life in general.

All of this will give you insight into yourself and arm you with information—empirical information—that will help you have the conversations you (and we) need to have.

That's what I want you to consider this book—a long-overdue conversation. First between you and me. Then between you and your family, your community, and your fellow Americans.

I want to help you *be who you are on purpose.*

I want to help you give yourself permission to live consistent with your beliefs and values and do so with pride and conviction. We Americans are a melting pot with many definitions of *who* we are and *what* we consider important. And that's great as long as embracing one's personal values doesn't infringe on the rights of others, or as long as there is no effort to cram a personal agenda down other people's throats. Living with differences can be both interesting and healthy.

Ultimately, though, I believe all change—namely societal change and global change—starts with the individual. It's like the story of the little boy who was pestering his father while he was trying to work. The father started to look for something that could distract his son for a while. He found a page in a magazine with a map of America. He ripped the page out and cut it into pieces. "You like puzzles," he said. "Here's some tape—see if you can put America back together." Thinking he had bought himself an hour or two of peace, he was surprised when his son came to him ten minutes later with a perfectly reassembled map of the United States. "How is that possible? You don't even know the map of the United States." The son said, "I don't know the map of America. But on the other side of the page you tore out there was a picture of a person. When I fixed the person, it also fixed the world."

That's why we're going to help you be who you are on purpose.

Because in the process, we're going to fix some of this divisiveness in our country.

Without the more than 330 million of us Americans, America is just a big landmass. What makes America "America" is *We the people*! You and me.

I believe we can recapture the American narrative and find a way to live in harmony. That is going to take some work, because I think there is a lot of "cramming" going on, a lot of hijacking of America's narrative by individuals and groups who are ignoring science and history and just making up a new reality. And they are *not* minding their own business. As my grandma used to say, "They've stopped preaching and gone to meddling."

Not everyone deserves a seat at the table we're building right now. Not every voice gets to be heard. There are prerequisites like facts, science, and a willingness to open your mind and maybe even change it. You good with that? Great. Let's work together and get this wonderful country back on track, starting right now.

Thanks for hearing me out. I wanted you to know precisely why I have written this book.

Phillip C. "Dr. Phil" McGraw, Ph.D.
Dallas, Texas
10/30/23

INTRODUCTION

We've Got Issues

POLL QUESTION

How often do you feel in control of your own life?

☐ Always

☐ Most of the time

☐ Sometimes

☐ Never

I love this country. I love it for what it offers and has offered to me and my family and most everyone I have ever known. I am proud to be an American. Is it a perfect country? No, of course not, not by a long shot, but neither are any of us. I guess there is a certain symmetry to that because as I say, we *are* this country!

There are parts of our history that are not proud. But there are things going on today that I find equally unnerving.

You are going to learn that this is all being driven by a small number of people who claim to be representing large segments of our society. I don't believe that is true.

I find myself waking up in the middle of the night deeply concerned about where we are collectively headed as a country. There is one thing that helps me get back to sleep. I believe all these activists, like so many who see things from only their own point of view, are committing a strategic error. I believe they have yelled so loud and so long and pushed so hard and so far that they have inadvertently awakened a sleeping giant. You. A member of what has, until now, been a massive group of Americans from every walk of life who shared the common value: "Live and let live." But everyone, individually and collectively, has a point where they "dig in their heels" and say, "Enough is enough and too much is too much."

Neither history, biology, nor the laws of nature can be rewritten just because someone *wishes* they were different. I said I would be transparent about my point of view from the start, and what I have just written is a big part of it: I do love America and I do respect facts.

Facts exist! Scientific results exist. They are, by definition, observable, measurable, and repeatable. You can't wish them away. There are scientific realities in physics, in chemistry, in biology, and other empirically defined fields. Use the scientific reality of simple gravity as your hypothetical test case. To follow this logic trail, just decide you hypothetically don't believe in, like, or want to have gravity anymore.

Then when you think you have sufficiently discarded, debunked, relabeled, and rallied support among fellow antigravity adherents, just live your convictions and take a giant step off a three- or four-story ledge and see what happens! Just stride right off the edge and see if your disdain for gravity and the number of adherents in the antigravity society you formed or the marches you organized against the National Science Foundation, or the science professor you attempted to blacklist because he or she continues to teach about gravity, make a tinker's damn bit of difference in the reality of how hard you faceplant. (Actually, do *not* do that. It would be idiotic, dangerous, and harmful, like a lot of other ideologies being peddled today—which is basically my point.)

It seems silly. You might think—if someone wants to go on living their antigravity life, what does their constant face-planting have to do with me? I want to be clear, *all of us* are involved whether we think so or not. Every one of us takes a position on everything happening in this country and in our lives of which we have any conscious awareness. As I said a minute ago: in this culture war, you don't have the luxury of being a noncombatant. *You cannot not choose.* Why? Because even not choosing is a choice.

I need to emphasize my point here because it is essential to grasping the entirety of this book: *You cannot not choose.* And by the way, you also cannot "unread" those words; you can't "unknow" that truth.

Think about this analogy: Picture yourself way out in the country. It is flat as a pancake, nothing but plowed fields. You can see for miles in every direction. Now imagine you come to a crossroads. You are standing right in the middle of the intersection, pondering, as you look at four wide, flat highways each headed in a different direction, north, south, east, and west.

You can go left, or you can go right. You can go straight ahead or reverse course and go back the way you came. Those would clearly seem to be your four choices. But there is a fifth choice. You can *choose* to not decide and just stand there in the middle of the intersection. Eventually, you'll get run over. That *is* the fifth choice, and it's the choice a lot of people are making—intentionally or unintentionally. Which is why I say *you cannot not choose, because not choosing is a choice.* Same deal here: Remaining silent *is* a choice. Deciding to not weigh in on a relevant issue *is* a choice. Having a conversation only with yourself *is* a choice.

All of us are either advancing, eliciting, allowing, or maintaining what is going on in our lives. I did not choose those words at random. These are the four ways in which you are playing a role regarding the toxicity in your life.

When I say "toxicity," I'm not talking about our politics, Democrats, or Republicans. I'm talking about our *culture, our values and beliefs, our family units, the building blocks upon which America has been structured.*

And I'm not just talking about the divisiveness we are experiencing. That's an *effect, not a cause.* I'm talking about the cause: a much broader, sustained attack on core values and principles. Principles that if not embraced and defended can spell the end of the country as we have known it.

That may sound overly dramatic, but think about it: What can you put on a list that is going on in America right now that you would never have dreamed possible? I won't share my full list just yet. But you can start your own. Why do *you* need a list? Because these people who are among us right now are trying to reframe reality not just in their own lives but for us all. I suppose it would be different if they were living like hermits in the woods and kept their bizarre ideologies to themselves. Unfortunately, that is not what's happening. They are pushing various unfounded ideologies in our schools and universities, the corporate world, on the internet, and anywhere else they can get an audience.

Did you ever think school board policy would require or support teachers and students purposefully conspiring to lie to parents, even by omission, about deeply important personal issues such as gender identity (or anything else for that matter)?

Whether you think they should or shouldn't inject themselves between a student and their parent, I do wonder where they find the time to pay attention to *anything* other than advancing the academic curriculum, the job for which they were hired, especially when the National Assessment of Educational Progress reports roughly 30 percent of fourth *and* eighth graders can't read at even the most basic level.[1] The US Department of Education and Literacy Inc. further reported that 19 percent of high school graduates can do no better![2]

And the tumble down the academic hillside is ongoing. In June 2023, results distributed by the National Center for Education Statistics (a branch of the Education Department) revealed that in 2022, math and reading scores for thirteen-year-olds had dropped another nine and four points, respectively. Math scores showed the biggest drop in fifty years. Scores declined across all age groups, including elementary students. And while the National Assessment of Educational Progress points out that US history scores for middle schoolers aren't too far from where they were when the first assessment was given in 1994, the harsh truth is that they are at the lowest level ever recorded.

Teachers, teachers' unions, and school boards must be 100 percent focused on academics and existing curriculums and not be distracted by the "virtue signaling" demanded by the tyrannical activists who use emotional extortion to get compliance. Do what we want or you will be labeled, picketed, targeted as a "hater," and boycotted. Absent this leverage, this would seem an easy decision, especially when those involved typically have no training beyond teaching. Teaching could not be more important. It is an honorable (and terribly underpaid) profession staffed by dedicated individuals, so very many of whom tell me they would like nothing better than to be allowed to teach rather than being drafted into an army of social justice warriors (SJW). My research over the last three years, admittedly anecdotal but with solid, published documentation, suggests the teachers' *unions* are the driving force behind many of the extreme social agenda changes to especially the elementary or lower school curriculums.

And when teachers are pushed to "get out of their lane" and into the psychosocial functioning of a student, they are often dealing with a child they may have just met and therefore have no firsthand experience or knowledge of that child's mental, emotional, social, familial, medical, or genetic predispositions. They are no more trained and prepared to engage in such sensitive developmental, self-image, and identity issues than they would be if they were asked to remove that same child's spleen during homeroom!

Or let's take a look at the justice system, which has clearly become so heavily influenced by an overly socially progressive agenda that way too many criminals—from misdemeanor offenders to repeat violent felons—are no longer properly held to account. Even blatant and repeat shoplifters are now often allowed to walk right into a store as if they were a normal customer, take what they want, and just stroll out the front door knowing they will not be so much as asked to "please don't do that." This now happens with such frequency that not just small "mom-and-pops" but huge brand, chain stores that deal in millions and millions of dollars of transactions daily are being forced out of business from the weight of the losses. What is seriously troubling is that a significant percentage of Gen Zers (twenty-five and under) *defend* the shoplifters, saying they have a right to take what is "rightfully theirs." Why? Because they maintain everyone is entitled to a certain standard of living as a basic human right!

If that wasn't enough, we have educators and academic historians rewriting history to misrepresent to your children what has transpired in this country's past. Tearing down statues and changing school names due to behavior that, while certainly unacceptable today, was much more mainstream two-hundred-plus years ago and, like it or not—factually *did* occur. Painful lessons were learned and now for reasons no one can satisfactorily explain to me, attempts are being made to bury those lessons.

Those are just a few examples on my mind, and I will share many more as we move forward. I realize you may have different priorities and areas of concern and these topics might not even make your top twenty. That's okay as long as we are thinking and both giving a voice to what does matter to us and our loved ones.

If these things or others that do bother you greatly are happening—and sadly, they are—the question we both have to ask ourselves is, What are we going to do about it?

At some level, we all have to know, standing by and allowing these kinds of things to happen in our society can't continue. We are blowing the world's most successful social experiment, the greatest opportunity mankind has ever created: a chance to live in, benefit from, and nurture a peaceful nation where we are truly free in every respect.

Since you cannot not choose, ask yourself: What choices am I making?

Are there things in your life, your family's life, your community, state, or nation that you shake your head about, complain to spouse or friends about, but when it comes down to it, take no action that has even a chance to result in change? If so, you may not be "intentionally advancing" the activists' agenda, but aren't you enabling it by creating space and time for it in your mind, heart, and even family? Aren't you allowing and maintaining it through your inaction or by telling someone what they want to hear, by publicly reciting the lie to escape their tyranny?

Apparently, in this country, we just can't stand success, because despite having a government that guarantees critically important freedoms, despite recognizing that many of our forebears fought and died to preserve, protect, and defend important individual freedoms and rights like free speech and self-governance, we have become so lost and misguided that *we*, not the government, are threatening and in some cases acting to *take those things away from each other*!

Sadly, free speech is a great example. The government is not violating that fundamental right, but, incredibly, we are trying to *muzzle each other*!

This insane behavior goes by a lot of names: "cancel culture," "character assassination," or "guilt by accusation"—all fueled by a mob mentality that is the stock in trade for the Tyrants of the Fringe and is hypercharged by an out-of-control internet (or perhaps more accurately a *weaponized* internet) with fake accounts used to harass people or "bot farms" that create hundreds or thousands of automated messengers to amplify a message and make it "look" legit and feel widespread.

This is so rampant, the majority of Americans now feel threatened and intimidated, afraid to speak up about troubling trends that are undeniably building momentum. Trends that I believe, when examined, any rational person *knows* make no sense and if tolerated will prove to be destructive.

People stand silent for fear of being targeted and bullied by the self-appointed arbiters of justice, worried that they may be ostracized by others (even though those others may even secretly agree with the person being bullied, but are afraid to say—demonstrating the psychodynamic characteristic of "defensive identification").

I can't help but wonder, when did so many Americans become afraid to stand up for each other and what's good and right? Social research, not just opinion, suggests that it occurred pretty recently.

From the 1950s to today, the percentage of Americans who don't feel free to express their views has *tripled*. That means we are moving backward. People feel less free to speak their minds today than they did almost seventy-five years ago! More than half of Americans say that they have held their tongue, that is, not spoken freely over the last year, because they were concerned about retaliation or harsh criticism.[3]

Eighty-four percent of Americans today say that the fear of retaliation or criticism causing people not to share their views is a serious problem. Is it because the internet—which didn't exist seventy-five years ago—allows us to be "called out" so easily by so many people? The ability to attack someone is now instantaneous, it is anonymous, and it is accessible by a bunch of "keyboard bullies."

Why am I choosing to write about this multi-front assault on our society, culture, families, and very way of life? And multi-front it is: free speech, paying people *not* to work, failing to enforce laws and maintain order in our cities, and many more to come. I'm writing about these issues and trends because while they may appear to be political, and may get talked about by politicians, they are fundamentally rampant, self-destructive psychosocial phenomena.

These are cultural, not political, issues that boil down to what people are willing to do, say, accept, and/or support in society. I'm writing about it because I see it, I *know* where it is headed, and I *refuse to choose to accept it.* I can, I should, and I feel like I must write about what's happening. I will not stand paralyzed in the middle of the intersection and watch as this insanity continues to barrel down the road at us. I *am* making a choice.

Do I think I have a big enough voice to stop the unfounded ideologies, the refusal to adhere to science, or the failure to commit to being a nation of laws? Of course not. Not a chance. But I believe *we* do. I believe together we can stand up, step up, and speak up against those things we believe will erode our country and our values, our families and futures.

The "live and let live" mass of Americans, the "we" alluded to above, I believe, has been pushed too far. I believe mainstream Americans can and are beginning to push back with a powerful message of self-determination and rejection of manipulation. The transgender "ideology" being so aggressively pushed by transgender activists, but not necessarily the transgender community as a whole, has been self-destructive, serving to mobilize the mainstream population against the transgender community. Many all across America, especially but not limited to parents, have objected to this conversation being forced into schools, saying that they are "sexualizing" children. They object to teachers getting involved in young students' personal lives, often to the exclusion of parents, and fight against transgender students using school bathrooms not consistent with the sex that appears on their birth certificate.

I feel a great sense of urgency because I believe there are many issues where mainstream America (that would be *you*) believes "enough is enough and too much is too much." When people are being criticized and made to feel guilty just for loving their country, imperfect as it may be, it's time *somebody* speaks up. It's time a lot of somebodies speak up. The people peddling what they are peddling may have the right to say it; they may have the right to publish it, broadcast it, even sell it. But we most certainly have the right to reject it. It is time to stand our ground, and start reclaiming the ground we've lost. For too long, from a psychological standpoint, I have felt like I'm tied to a chair, watching a child play with a live grenade. Well, I'm finally working my wrists free. Maybe it's been too long in coming, but the time is always right to do what's right. For me, that time is now and what's right is writing this book.

I know how I feel, and I am betting a lot of you feel the same way. But to be entirely honest, this is not so much about feelings as it is about facts. People are always telling me how they "feel." I get it. That's the line of work I'm in. But when it comes to the kind of things I'm talking about, I don't really care how you feel. I barely care how I feel!

In the following pages, I'm going to hand you a product you can *use*, to stand up, step up, and speak up, be your authentic self, and save our country in the process. I predict that a lot of your suspicions, your gut-level instincts, are going to be validated by verifiable, hard-edged data. The data proves that so much of what is being so sanctimoniously crammed down your throat has absolutely no basis in reality, *no supporting evidence* whatsoever! It is fiction, fantasy espoused by people who *wish* it were true because that is how *they feel things should* be. Like I said, somebody needs to challenge the toxic mentality currently overrunning American culture, the destructive agendas undermining America, and stand up to the bullies pushing it all.

The attacks being leveled on the American family and the American way of life do not appear to be random. Some of the activist agendas just seem so focused on disrupting the very heart of our existence as to be intentional. These agendas are ideologically, morally, and psychosocially "nuclear."

You start tampering with American's children, their family and the ability to navigate peacefully through this life, and you risk awakening that giant I keep talking about—that powerful and dedicated mass of Americans of which you and I are proudly a part. Maybe we have been a relatively passive group ideologically, but that should never be confused with weakness and most definitely not confused with being unprincipled. Pushed to the brink value-wise, with our existence threatened, we will not stay silent, will not cower. We will rear back on our hind legs, roar, and fight for who we are and who we care about and what we believe and value. Look no further than any heated school board meeting.

We are at that point. Those seeking to push agendas that continue to divide this country are about to see, feel, and experience American resolve.

One pattern I see occurring all too often that has me beyond concerned is what I see happening with what can only be described as "woke" and, in my opinion, seriously uninformed and misguided university professors and even administrators who are supposedly conducting courses on a defined subject matter, but instead are arrogantly pressing their personal, cultural, and political agendas onto young, impressionable, captive audiences.

From positions of assigned authority, paid by our tax dollars in many cases, they are pushing their own personal belief systems and often criticizing such qualities as masculinity, ambition, and the drive for success. Rather than identifying "toxic masculinity," they label masculinity itself as toxic. They teach that being competitive is predatory and therefore a bad trait. They preach that aggressively pursuing a goal is gauche. These "educators" pushing their own personal beliefs rather than empirically supported positions hold that seeking financial success is unenlightened. They teach that we should all strive for equality of outcome because all humans deserve the same result in life independent of their contribution. They teach that words can cause physical harm, harm that people need to be protected from. I find these ideologies masquerading as "academic content" arrogant and appalling.

I have seen and heard of these topics dominating classes that were not sociology or economics or anything related to psychosocial dynamics. What gives these "professors" the right to professionally hobble young men (in particular) who are going to have to enter a highly competitive world and have to provide for their future family? What gives them the right to teach our talented young people exactly 100 percent how the world does *not work*? And where will these fairy-tale professors, who have probably never had a job where they had to "put up or shut up," be later when the rent is due and the child of that student needs braces? I can tell you where: gone! You won't be able to find them with both hands and a flashlight! Lots of opinions, plenty of misguided advice, but no accountability.

I know I shouldn't be surprised, because this has been going on in academia for decades. Postmodernism (which I'll discuss in the upcoming chapter) and the idea of subjective truth, identity politics, Marxism (a constant war between the classes): all these ideas have blossomed and cross-pollinated in the academic greenhouse—where they could flourish without having to survive the droughts, snows, and storms of the real world. But the seeds have scattered far beyond that greenhouse and sprung up in entertainment, media, and corporate America. And these ideologies don't leave much room for alternatives. My belief is that it is this kind of mindset being pushed on our young generation in ultraliberal university settings where shouting down speakers who dare to present a different point of view is clear evidence of the closed-minded, sanctimonious self-righteousness that has led to some of the abuses whistleblowers have disclosed recently. This has been particularly true of the social media giants that have decided *they* get to decide what you and I see and hear. A terrible, totalitarian-sounding threat to our way of life, in my humble opinion.

But there is an alternative way to live our lives and approach the challenges and opportunities of our world: self-determination. The belief that we create our own experience in this world. Yes, it is true some of us start from further behind than others. Some of us are born on third base and recognize our blessings. Some of us are born on third base and think we hit a triple. No matter where we were born—third base, dugout, or dumpster—we all, through our choices, behaviors, efforts, and attitudes, determine the outcome of our lives. When we lose that belief, when parents fail to instill it, when schools fail to teach it, we lose one of the key elements that makes America America.

It used to be, when I had a hiring choice between someone who graduated from college and someone who didn't, I would choose the college graduate because I knew something about them I didn't know about the nongraduate. It was not because they knew more or were smarter, but because to me, a college degree meant that candidate had learned how to navigate a tough world. Among other things, they had figured out how to set and meet a multiyear objective, and how to get along with some jerk professors along the way. I'm not saying that the person without the college degree couldn't do those things; it was just that I *didn't know* that about them. But I can't say that anymore. Because the young men and women college graduates I meet now have been softened, corrupted in their thinking to the point that they can be wounded by words, sabotaged, and ideologically seduced by a socialistic fiction that history has repeatedly proven to be so unqualifiedly disastrous.

Another example of what I'm talking about is the phenomenon of "quiet quitting" that we have seen occurring in the last few years. This again is something that I don't believe would be happening if it were not for the internet giving oxygen to a sentiment that a small handful of people might have shared before technology allowed bad ideas to spread far, wide, and fast. Quiet quitting, as described and discussed on social media platforms by thousands upon thousands of young people in the workforce, is a concerted strategy to, for lack of a better term, just "go through the motions" at work. Don't do a single thing more than you're asked or required to do. Don't offer to pitch in or help out on something that's not directly in your job description. Don't go that extra mile to get ahead.

Now, I will grant you there are certainly a lot of exploitive bosses out there. By and large, however, I think workplaces tend to be pretty collaborative. These people deciding to do just the bare minimum are going to get just that in terms of their review, salary considerations, and longevity. They will deny themselves the mentorship and time with leaders that the occasional late night or early morning will provide. When the public proponents of quiet quitting decide it's time to get busy and put their lives on track, I believe they will rue the day that they created a permanent record for every HR department they ever interacted with to review and judge. It just doesn't sound like a very smart or promising life approach to me. But, when you misinform and coddle a generation, these are the types of things you get.

These young people are so greatly weakened and misguided it can literally ruin their lives because they simply can't function in the real world. If you're reading closely right now, you might say: Pick a side, Dr. Phil! Is it the professors indoctrinating the students? Or are the professors being intimidated by the coddled students? The answer is both. People in a bad environment *can* bring out the worst in each other. Either way you spin it, the results are disastrous. It's shocking that students who are the product of concierge parents, and who then get coddled by "woke and enlightened" but clueless professors, are not turning out to be high performers!

Instead of properly preparing a generation of amazingly intelligent, capable young people, students are now so thin-skinned they come to believe that words can actually hurt them or that when they fail a class it's the teacher's fault. We're looking at a generation of young people taught to believe it is the world's, their employer's, or their institution's job to get along with them rather than learning when they enter an organization that it is *their job* to get along with everyone else and to work hard to earn respect and success.

This concerns me because I believe this attitude—whether it is specifically espoused by asleep-at-the-switch professors getting out of their lane and sabotaging impressionable students or a product of the institutions of higher learning having "sold out" to an anti-merit-based agenda—leaves students fundamentally unprepared. It seems hypocritical to me that these colleges and universities sell a supposedly elite education to give graduates an "edge" but then adopt the rhetoric that having an edge somehow violates someone else's right to a dignified human experience.

Ignoring the very clear lesson (one that has been proven time and again throughout history and around the world) that experiments in socialism do not work over any sustained amount of time, the idea that we should have equality of outcome regardless of the quality of the input doesn't even make common sense. Even in theory, it only works until (to paraphrase Margaret Thatcher) you run out of other people's money.

People learn what they live. If they live a life of entitlement, if they learn that you can make more money not working than by working, guess what? You are going to have a lot of people who just can't see the sense in working.

This, by the way, *is happening*. I'm talking about able-bodied, able-minded people who can and should be pulling their own weight. We are disincentivizing an entire generation of working-age people, and the fallout is so massive that there aren't enough trees in this world to make enough paper to write a book fully describing it.

Among other things, we're talking about a group of people—millions of Americans—who are highly depressed, lacking in self-esteem, lacking in goals and passion for life. They have become dependent, and when the money runs out (which is inevitable) they will be ill-equipped to get back into the swing of things. This is all going to hit the fan sooner than later, and shame on the shortsighted, self-serving idealists who, unwilling to confront or prepare for reality, are ruining these people's lives. You don't have to wonder if this kind of mindset is working or not working. Look at the levels of depression, anxiety, and loneliness among this generation. I would argue that some of that comes from the impact of cheating them out of the pride of setting and achieving goals, the reward of overcoming obstacles and being able to say, "I did that. I worked hard, I persevered, and I'm proud of accomplishing something of importance." They have been denied the feeling of "I'm starring in my own life!" Instead we are seeing psychological pain and a lack of personal gratification.

Our government certainly isn't helping by handing out free money. That doesn't work. When you give people substantial amounts of money for an extended period of time with no prerequisite of performance, added value, or any expectations whatsoever, you are conditioning them to expect to be "taken care of." During the two-year COVID-19 quarantine it has been reported that from all sources (including stimulus checks, extended unemployment payments, the expanded Child Tax Credit, and more) the government gave out $5.5 trillion with no expectations. It has also been reported that $4.4 trillion of it went into savings accounts, clearly indicating that 80+ percent of that money was not needed, yet it was paid out anyway.

Anyone who knows the first thing about behavioral economics will tell you that you are paralyzing the workforce when people can make as much money not working as they can working. I sat back and shook my head as I watched our government, which was already sitting on roughly $30 trillion in debt, start distributing another

matter how much you may want to escape accountability,
how much you may want to sit on the sidelines, you are
me. And when you make a choice you own everything that
long with it.

en I talk about the "tyranny of the fringe," I'm talking about
who often ignore or seriously distort empirical science because,
me personal or ideological reason, they don't *want* something to
rue. These are people (more specifically, activists) who simply
ide to redefine something like biology. And sadly, this is happen-
g at every level of education.

> en I talk about the
> anny of the fringe,"
> talking about people
> who often ignore or
> eriously distort empirical
> science because, for some
> personal or ideological
> reason, they don't *want*
> something to be true.

A lot of people who are getting a free ride or who want to be validated for just showing up will not like me saying any of this out loud. But I say it with the confidence that they will love me later if I somehow cause them to learn to actually cope, compete, and survive in the real world. And even if they don't come around, I want them to at least have had the truth available.

Fortunately, I am not afflicted with the need to be loved by strangers. (I suspect that is going to come in as handy as a pocket on a shirt when this book gets out there.)

If you don't see a problem with any of the "reverse incentive system" I just mentioned, if you think the real world is not a meritocracy where hard work, added value, and talent should win out the vast majority of the time, my question to you is, "What are you pretending not to know?"

The *real world* is very competitive. And if we don't get the current (and every) generation in this country ready to compete in areas that matter—instead of figuring out how many ways they can cry victim

$5.5 trillion! The only sense I co□
to cover up for the gross mismana□
quarantine that wiped out many sma□
of many hardworking Americans. Un□
two wrongs don't make a right.

It doesn't take an economist, a behaviora□
gist to figure out that if you create a system whe□
money by not working than they can by work□
good they're going to stay on the couch. What re□
all the bureaucrats with puzzled looks on their faces□
began to open up after two years, they found out the □
paralyzed. I wonder if that had anything to do with the□
were paying the people who kept it moving more money □
than to work? Time to get out the mirror and see if someb□
writing on my forehead, because it sure looks to me like we are □
ing behavior *we do not want: Stay home, don't work, get free mone*□

We're seeing cities adopt the insane mindset that contorts r□
to say that the criminal is the real victim, and therefore there sho□
be few to no consequences for criminal actions. One of the things □
believe deeply and say often is that when you choose the behavior,
you choose the consequences. When that ceases to be the case, we
have *really lost our way.* Already I have hit some big points that, when
you internalize and apply them, will make you extremely potent as a
change agent:

➤ We cannot reward bad behavior.

➤ You cannot *not* choose. Even deciding not to make a
  choice is by definition *a choice.*

➤ When you choose the behavior, you choose the consequences.

➤ We must deal with facts, not fiction.

or be carried—they and all those depending on them later will be "chewed up and spit out."

As I write this, the country is debating something that recently happened at Stanford Law School, the latest in a series of episodes where speakers on campus have been shouted down and hounded out of town. Stanford's chapter of the Federalist Society, a conservative legal organization, invited Judge Stuart Kyle Duncan to talk about his court.

Judge Duncan's politics are no secret. He argued before the Supreme Court against the constitutionality of same-sex marriage. He's defended the bathroom bill in North Carolina that prohibits transgender students from using the bathroom that corresponds to their gender identity. Agree with him or disagree with him, he's a judicial force to be reckoned with.

Or, if you're a Stanford law student, shouted down. Because when he got up to speak, students immediately began shouting things like "You're not welcome here, we hate you" and "You have no right to speak here." After about ten minutes of this abuse, Judge Duncan asked for help restoring order from the Stanford administrators who were there.

Stanford Law School's dean for diversity, equity, and inclusion (DEI) got up and read a statement that basically sided with the hecklers, saying that Judge Duncan's work had caused "harm" to students.[4] Duncan wasn't able to finish his talk, and America got to see what I would argue is a dangerous new form of political power: the "heckler's veto," where the loudest voice (as we'll discuss later) can drown out the voices we would benefit from hearing.

And while the dean talked about harm, there was already a different type of harm going on at Stanford Law School. As one student described it, "an academic environment with two loud camps, one aligning with far-right politics, one aligning with far left. In between, where most students can be found: silence. There's little room for nuance. If you're not overtly one of 'us,' then you're assumed to be one of 'them' . . . expressing nuance about certain matters—whether on Israel or policing—is essentially taboo for someone who doesn't want to invite social ostracizing."[5]

So, what did these students accomplish by shouting down a judge? Two things. First, they denied everyone—themselves included—the chance to understand the judge's arguments, which would be a useful thing to know if they ever wanted a chance to refute them.

Second, they limited their own career prospects. Several judges have already announced they will refuse to hire clerks from Stanford Law School.[6]

The question I focus on *every day*, the question that has compelled me since I was twelve years old, is "Why do people do what they do and don't do what they don't do?" Understanding the answer to that question is critical to understanding human behavior at its most basic level.

The family unit in America is the backbone of our society. It is the fundamental building block of our culture. And as I said, this is a book about culture, not politics. Politicians come and go. They talk a lot and do a little. Maybe that's a good thing. I personally feel safer when there is "gridlock" in Washington, DC. Heck, our system is actually designed for gridlock, for not much to get done—regardless of who is in charge. In that sense, it's working like a charm.

We are, more or less, a fifty-fifty nation. In recent history, Republicans have been in charge about as much as Democrats. But culture, the "collective personality" we create together, is what determines the outcomes of our society.

I'm very worried that what is going on in our culture right now—everything I'm talking about and more—is threatening our society. American values, the *core family unit*, and our very way of life. To the extent possible, I am going to identify exactly what it is, in my opinion, they are trying to destroy.

I say "to the extent possible" because when it gets really outrageous, for example telling us what words we can no longer use (a list that would be too long for Einstein to remember and with reasoning too convoluted for him to decipher), the activists often don't sign their demands with their own names! They tell us what words we are expected *to* use. They dictate it, but they don't "own it." The *they* is an identifiable group, even when their members don't step forward. Instead it is signed off by the "Committee to Improve Human Harmonious Interaction" or some such lofty, self-aggrandizing crap. It's like that old joke that business meetings demonstrate that none of us is as dumb as *all* of us. Put a bunch of well-meaning eggheaded people together to produce an anonymous report, and more often than not you'll get some monumental stupidity.

But I am also going to make every effort to identify for you *why they are doing it*, so that you can be better prepared to understand their *payoff*. Trust me, there is one. People don't generally do things, in pattern, if they aren't getting *something* out of it. That *something* can be constructive or destructive. And in this case, we're talking toxic.

I want you to keep in the back of your mind these two basic explanatory, motivational concepts: envy and selfishness.

I am confident you will hear what I have to say, weigh it carefully, challenge every position if you are so inclined, fact-check me until you are "blue in the face," as my mother used to say, and then make up your *own mind*.

Lately, too many people seem more focused on winning arguments than solving problems. Maybe we have made the mistake of taking for granted this fabulous, amazing country we have been so blessed to live in, work in, and raise our families in.

Big mistake. Huge, monumental mistake.

If you've listened to me for any amount of time, I'll bet you've heard me say, "The best predictor of future behavior is relevant past behavior."

If you want to know what is most likely going to happen today, take a look at what happened yesterday. In America, good things just happen. That is, they happen, until they don't, until something significant comes along to "disrupt the flow."

Our issues have gotten in the way of our progress. And so we're living in an America that's been disrupted.

I will be asking you a series of questions throughout this book, one or two at the top of each chapter. Those questions are part of a national poll I have designed and administered in the hopes of helping you understand where you are as you progress through the book.

At the end of each chapter, I will reveal how thousands of people nationwide responded to that chapter's specific question. There are no right or wrong answers, and no one answer is better than another. I offer the data purely for your information. It will allow you to see how many others share or differ from your thinking and experiences. It is up to you to decide what the data says about your frame of mind and that of your fellow Americans.

For example, I started this chapter by asking how often you feel in control of your own life. As I was writing this book, I surveyed nearly 1,200 *Dr. Phil* viewers. As you might expect, the "sample" closely tracked the population makeup of the people who have followed me for the last couple of decades: more women than men, more conservative than liberal, slightly older and whiter than the population overall—but a very diverse group in terms of income and educational level. Again, these findings aren't intended to tell you what you should think. They simply tell you where you stand. And you can decide if that's where you want to be.

POLL RESPONSE

How often do you feel in control of your own life?

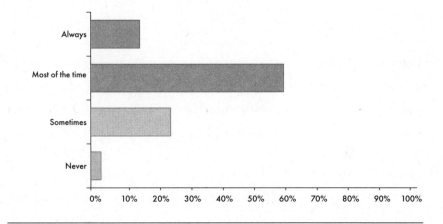

CHAPTER 1

The Price and Consequences
of Disruption

POLL QUESTION

How concerned are you that "fringe groups" are trying to
hijack and displace core values, scientific findings, and an
unbiased view of history in America?

☐ Very

☐ Somewhat

☐ Not very

☐ Not at all

You hear the word *disruption* a lot. But I don't mean that word, *disruption*, in the way that tech inventors do when they talk about how some new invention is going to change your life. I'm talking about how America's values, the core principles upon which this country has been built, have been toxically disrupted. When things you once just *counted on*, things that in America were *no-brainers*, start falling by the wayside, like that America would have the best education system, the best health care system, the greatest chance to get ahead (social mobility), *heck, the best postal system*: it's time to start asking hard questions and paying careful attention to red flag warnings. We *all* need to start asking, Why? Is it some kind of natural evolution? Is it some kind of societal decay? Or maybe it is not natural at all.

Think of all the things that dominate the headlines, subjects we spend time talking about, debating, and fighting over instead of focusing on issues that really matter. And while we've been investing that time and energy because the advocates, who are organized and loud, demand it, we have lost time and energy focusing on issues that impact the other 99 percent of Americans. Both have a place on the agenda, but we need to have a sense of proportion.

But do we? Or have we had our primary national narrative hijacked by special interest groups focused only on their self-referential agendas? Have we failed to pay attention to the important issues that impact all Americans?

I don't want to give you my opinion. Let's look at some facts and see how the people we are paying to manage trillions of our tax dollars (a projected $4.71 trillion for 2023) and many of the things that touch our lives are doing. As I'm writing this section of the book a notification popped up on my computer screen that there was just a bipartisan vote to lift the debt ceiling above $34.1 trillion! Think about that for a minute, maybe two. Do you ever wonder *who America owes over $34 trillion*? Maybe the most shocking element of the whole thing is they called the bill to raise the limit, wait for it . . . "THE FISCAL RESPONSIBILITY ACT"! If you are not insulted and outraged right now, one of us is a fool. Our elected officials had to go into a room and decide, "We and everyone who came before us have put this country in the most irresponsible situation imaginable, and even though we're bringing in $4.71 trillion in tax revenue and plan to spend $5.8 trillion this year alone, we're good with the fact that we're just digging ourselves deeper into debt. So, let's call it the Fiscal RESPONSIBILITY Act. People just read headlines, not details, and that way every time we talk about it what comes out of our mouths are the words 'Fiscal' and 'Responsibility.' It will work. We will throw it right by them." Another example of twisting a definition and then sailing right along.

Our debt is over seven times our tax revenue and we keep looking for ways to give people free money, but if we are spending that much more than what we make, we must be doing great across the board, right? Let's take a look at the facts.

America is home to the greatest medical advances in the world. Yet would it surprise you to learn that the First World country where a woman is most likely to die in childbirth is none other than America?[1]

That's right: America is first in *maternal mortality* rate among the twenty high-income countries monitored.

In fact, the babies don't fare any better. There are fifty countries in the world that have a lower infant mortality rate than America. But we are first in some areas.

America is first in suicide rate among the G7 countries.

America is first in drug-related deaths among thirteen international peer countries. Two hundred and seventy-seven lives lost per million residents.[2]

America is first in health care costs compared to eleven international peer counties, but has the *lowest health care performance*.

America is first in motor vehicle deaths.

America is first in killings by police.

We are second worldwide for depression, fourth for murder, and sixth for incarceration rate. There are fifty-two countries that have a higher life expectancy.

Oh, but don't worry too much, because we're less likely to realize how bad that is because we've dropped to twenty-seventh in the world in math[3] and 45 million Americans are functionally illiterate and read below a fifth-grade level.[4]

The next time you hear a crowd chanting, "We're number one!" the sad truth is that we are number one, but in ways that aren't exactly cause for celebration.

We should all hear alarms going off when societal building blocks like education and mental health, solidly defined and time-tested principles and traditions like marriage and family unity, and even scientific facts and biological truths are treated like outdated and irrelevant news. When values and definitions as clear and fundamental as right and wrong are undercut and even mocked, we should all be concerned. We need to react behaviorally by prioritizing those fundamental things in our lives to ensure they are preserved.

If fringe factions, absent any rationale other than self-referential desire (by that I mean something, no matter how toxic or dangerous it may be, is important only to a small group of people), start to attack institutions as critical as the educational system, freedom of speech, the right to ask a question or express disagreement, self-determination, law enforcement, human rights, property rights, respect for science, reward for hard work, accountability, due process for the accused, the entire judiciary system, then we're beyond alarm-bell time. It is "call to action" time. Consider this book that call to action—because all of the above are being targeted.

When your children are advancing grade to grade but not getting a real education, it is time for action. If you are a parent, it is time to assert those rights and find out what is happening with your child. This is a big deal, huge. The quality of their education is powerfully linked to their future quality of life. Fight for them now. You are paying for that education with your tax dollars; if they cannot even read a menu, you are getting ripped off, and your child will pay the price. The mismanagement of COVID-19 may well have created an education and developmental gap from which they will never recover if not addressed (more on that in the chapter on the need to consistently test rationality of thought). But you are your child's advocate and the system doesn't have one minute to waste in nurturing your child. If they are spending time on *anything* else, your respectfully expressed objections need to be heard.

If you ask a good-faith question about almost anything affecting your life, and you expect a respectful, responsive answer, but instead you are attacked *just* for posing a question, or you go so far as exercising your First Amendment right to express a dissenting opinion and you are now defamed as a "hater" targeted for "cancellation," it is time for action.

If two-hundred-plus years of meritocracy in society is now considered somehow a conspiracy, and those who expect a hard day's work for a fair wage are considered oppressors, it is time for action.

When violent offenders are returned to the streets without regard for an innocent and unprepared public because *their* rights are being infringed. When store owners are being forced to close because of rampant uncontrolled theft.

When entire cities have been overtaken by homeless encampments or street mobs, this is an America Disrupted and it is time to get involved, a time for action.

All of a sudden, relevant past behavior is no longer predicting our future. When criticism of traditional American values, like respect for family and hard work, seems to be bending our culture, our policy, and our politics (even when there is no empirical data to support such criticism), it is time for action.

I can summarize a large part of this "call to action," this absolute moral imperative, a dictate of pure reason, in one sentence: the "we" I have been talking about can no longer be silent.

Do you ever wonder *why* small pockets of society seem able to control the narrative, to take center stage? They are able to do it for at least two reasons:

1. They identify a specific cause to rally around (real or imagined): educational agenda, racism, transgender issues, discrimination, fill in the blank.

2. They define a specific enemy. Someone or some group, company, or entity to target, boycott, picket, cancel, or complain about in a concentrated way. That attracts attention. Meanwhile, the majority of people who have no interest in any of these fights are content to remain on the sidelines. Maybe they're too busy working and keeping the world moving along. They have no interest in declaring enemies, no "rally location" identified or an assigned arrival time. No social media hashtag to express the fact that they want no part in the melee. The result is that the small seem large and the large seem *absent*!

As you've probably figured out by now, those "ifs" I mentioned are not hypothetical and you *do have rally points*. The "ifs" are a reality. And I could list many, many more ifs and red flags. These are not subtle signs. If you look at them all together, the red flags are about as obvious as a Navy signalman on the deck of an aircraft carrier frantically waving off an errant pilot. The future is getting bleaker and bleaker. If, If, If. *If* is the middle of the word *life*. You don't want to let yours get corrupted by a bunch of people who pretend science is, well, just irrelevant.

Nothing is immune from these history-ignoring and make-it-up-as-you-go-along "woke mobs."

This "woke mob" openly adheres to what is called "postmodernistic thinking." Under this definition, modernism was about having conversations based on objective truth, and geared toward maximizing progress. But with postmodernism, it's all about ideology.[5] It's a form of "self-referential" thinking that says that if it is important to me, it doesn't matter whether it is supported by science or not.[6] Common targets of postmodern criticism: science (which they openly mock), objective reality, morality, human nature, reason, language, and social progress. Reread those last few sentences, because your commonsense mind probably rejected them. But I am dead serious. These people actually brag about criticizing reality *and* science and just make up their own beliefs.

Still can't wrap your head around it? Here's one famous example, called the "Sokal Hoax." A physics professor named Alan Sokal decided to submit a scholarly article that "physical reality" isn't actually real—it's just a social and linguistic construct. He said that concepts like pi and gravity needed to be understood more on the grounds of social context, and he referred to the scientific method as the "so-called" scientific method. And a journal of cultural studies published it! It was total nonsense!

Pi is 3.14, no matter who you are. Sure, gravity is holding you down—but not economically or socially!

The type of people who fell for this hoax are the ones yelling the loudest and to whom we are mistakenly giving the most attention. That is who we are passively allowing to control the narrative in so many areas of our current society. They *know* they are making it up in order to fit their current agenda. They *make things up*. I am not that brazen *or* creative. This would be a great place to please fact-check me, because I wish I was wrong. But I'm not. You don't need to take my word for it. Go read about postmodernistic thinking. I'll even put a link for you in the footnotes.* Here is another example: if you dare talk about the role of the man in the family (leader, teacher, protector, and provider), someone is apt to step up and label you a misogynist at best. At worst, you're a hater, a mouth-breathing Neanderthal! Not just because you're describing a traditional role but because you used the "binary" term *man*. Am I seeing red? You bet and so should you.

---

* https://theconversation.com/explainer-what-is-postmodernism-20791.

Forces are in play, and our apathy, in many cases our fears, but in all cases our inaction and our wrongheaded thinking have enabled, empowered, even invited this disruption to occur. It is showing up in our schools, our universities, our most important companies, our books, and even in the dictionary.* They're sending us into uncharted and dangerous territory. It is time for action.

We simply must "get real" with ourselves and with each other. I am not prepared to watch this great country be driven off a cliff by a collection of loud, irrational radicals only to say, as the ground is approaching fast, "I should have said something, I should have done something." It is time we come together, unite, and take action. The first thing we have to do is acknowledge what is happening because, as I have often said, you can't change what you don't acknowledge.

If you have been shaking your head silently on the sidelines, you should be asking yourself why. Maybe you don't feel like anyone would listen if you *did* speak up.

Or maybe you feel like speaking up would put a target on your back—that you'd be labeled a "hater" or "fill-in-the-blank phobic."

By the way, this is one of the oldest and most desperate tactics in a debate, argument, or disagreement. If one side is losing a debate because the opponent is quoting some of those pesky damn demonstrable truths or objectively verified scientific facts and the other side has *none*, they just pivot and attack your character.

---

* Consider the case of the word *literally*—which is supposed to mean word-for-word true. If you are literally dying, then we should expect you to be dead in the near future. If you are literally starving, we would expect a doctor to look at you and say, "This person needs nutrition supplements, stat!" For a long time, people have misused *literally* to mean "figuratively," for emphasis. But now, instead of encouraging people to use the right word, with the right meaning, the Merriam-Webster and Cambridge dictionaries have basically thrown in the towel, and have said that *literally* no longer has to mean literally. People who can't use the right word have successfully gaslit us all into accepting the wrong word. It's a small thing, but a large symbol of what's going wrong.

If you think back to the playground you might remember the biting, "Yeah, well your mother wears army boots!" Little did I know as a fifth grader "out arguing" Michael by the tetherball poles that his personal attack on my dear, sweet mother would be no different from the current lowbrow mindset of today's postmodern "cancel culture."

Personal attacks on those who express different views are rampant. Unable to refute your logic, they label you. A personal insult is the death rattle of a reasoned debate, and we're hearing more and more of them every day.

And this is scary, because I'm guessing that the last thing in the world you or most people who have had their character assassinated are is a mean-spirited hater. Unless of course you accept the new definition of *hater*, which seems to be that you dare to disagree with some self-serving loudmouth.

In fact, I would hazard a guess that you're the opposite—you're full of love. Love for your family, community, and love for your country. That love is not naïve or unsophisticated. It's hopeful and dedicated and you shouldn't apologize for it, not for a minute.

Know Who You Are and *Own It*

How do we find the strength to push back? How do we overcome the behavioral paralysis, the fear of backlash should we make waves? Instead of taking our lives for *granted*, we fill our hearts and minds and fuel our lives with *gratitude* and a spirit of being a giver rather than a taker. I choose not to be motivated by guilt. I do not feel guilty for having healthy children, yet I have compassion and have worked to help those who do not. I do not feel guilty that my family has been happy and intact for forty-seven years or that my parents had been married for fifty-plus years when my father passed away. I have empathy for those who do not share that lived experience. I do not feel guilty for being white and well educated and financially stable. I don't need to feel guilty to feel compelled to help those who are none of those things—but I will do so in a way that the social sciences have taught me has the greatest chance of helping them break down barriers. Simply put, that is by reembracing the oft-cited distinction between the "hand up" and the "handout."

This isn't some new discovery. It's the age-old wisdom contained in the Chinese proverb "Give a man a fish and you feed him for a day. Teach a man to fish and you feed him for a lifetime."

Now, it's easy to tell people to pull yourself up by your bootstraps. But I fully recognize that some people don't have boots. Those who are none of the things I am fortunate to be deserve the boots: the better schools, better equipment, better-trained teachers, more community support and transitional help to get them into higher-paying jobs and careers. They need tools and an opportunity to use them. They need the inspiration to believe in themselves as well as healthy role models who get involved in their lives. What they don't need is free government money with no expectations. You do not solve money problems with money. They do not need standards lowered: that diminishes them and it weakens all of us. Put another way, you do not make your candle burn brighter by blowing out the candles of others. Aspiring to burn brightly *with* them is a straighter line to victory, for all of us. I have more to say about why I believe this— and why I get that it is easier said than done—in our chapter on the dangerous temptation of victimization when we discuss the work of the iconic Pastor Ward, who leads Insight Church, located outside of Chicago, and wrote a powerful book called *Zero Victim: Overcoming Injustice with a New Attitude.*

There are those out there who want me to feel guilty for being me and you to feel guilty for being you. But I simply do not and will not feel guilty for being me. I celebrate my blessings and work to help others in effective ways. The difference between winners and losers is that winners do things losers do not want to do. Guilt plays no part. Coercion plays no part. I've had many hills to climb and some still tower before me. For the most part, with hard work, persistence, resolve, and—I readily admit and fully recognize—more help along the way than I can even begin to tell you about in these pages, I've climbed a lot of hills.

So can others.

We all need help, but no one, absolutely no one else, can climb them for us.

Premise number one is that we have to be who we are *on purpose*! More about that later, but it means taking ownership. Give yourself permission to feel good, to consciously acknowledge who you choose to be, who you are, and what you are making and/or allowing to happen around you. Own you!

In the following pages, we're going to work through who you want to be—as an individual and collectively as a society—purposefully, head-on.

Just so I'm fully transparent, my starting position is this: I am grateful to be an American. I love America so much I don't have to be defensive about its shortcomings, which are many. I love it, flaws, fallacies, and all. Do I want America to be better as a country? Of course I do. There isn't space to make a thorough "to-do" list or probably even a "category" list. I just do not think we need to tear our country down or dishonor it in order to fix it. That just works to the advantage of our enemies. We are all Americans and should be proud while we work on getting better. I stand for the National Anthem. I put my hand over my heart to honor our flag. I am grateful to our men and women in uniform as well as our veterans. I think we should help those among us who are unable to help themselves. I could go on, but you get the picture.

How would you answer the same question regarding your "starting position"?

Let's Define Our Terms

I want to be clear about a few concepts we're talking about here. You've seen the word *woke*. I described it briefly above, but it has become so important and you hear it in your daily life all the time. So let me carefully define what my social science researchers put together from a thorough review of the current and historical literature. I strongly suspect it will make you the only one in the room who actually knows what you're talking about when the term comes up. The term has actually been around for a long time. Being "woke" was originally intended to describe people with a heightened awareness of social issues. To be "woke" meant to be enlightened about challenges facing the less fortunate, or, as a partial list of examples, those sensitized to dealing with racism, sexism, ableism, and homophobia. A new understanding about all sorts of human issues. There's certainly nothing wrong with that, about learning new things or understanding new things.

But somewhere along the line "wokeness" stopped being about awareness and started being an agenda. Specifically, the agenda of identity politics and an almost Marxist message: that the world is made up of oppressors and the oppressed, and you're on one side or the other. As a result, *woke* has now been redefined by the conduct of some (fewer than you might think, but well funded, well organized, and very loud) who betray its former meaning. It is now best characterized as a badge of political and cultural righteousness, by people making up new rules. It has been weaponized many times by misguided, self-righteous, sanctimonious activists running a toxic agenda fueled by a "mob mentality." It has been said that "power corrupts and absolute power corrupts absolutely." In many cases, these activists have "absolute power" because nobody is willing to hold them to account. Targeted individuals or organizations fear the ramifications of fighting back, lacking the audacity to question the intentions or actions of their attacker. It's like the old saying: Don't get in a mud-wrestling match with a pig. You get dirty and the pig likes it. There's no winning a fight with a woke activist, because they want the fight; that's why they picked it in the first place! Your reputation gets dirtied, and they like it because it brings attention to their cause.

Of course, the real damage is that once weaponized, *woke* has become the opposite of what it used to mean. Instead of greater understanding, it's about putting on a performance that *prevents* greater understanding. In *this context* that's what I'm talking about: the sort of performative righteousness that provides more heat than light.[7]

I also make several references to what I call the "live and let live" mass of Americans. I also said I believe that, once awakened, "we" can be a powerful cultural force to bring this country back to the core values that it has been built on. Collectively "we" can have amazing influence!

I want to be clear: I'm talking about culture, not politics. But there is a good analogy to what I'm saying that is undeniable whether you are a Democrat or a Republican. I'm talking about what is sometimes referred to as the "silent majority."

According to journalist Taegan Goddard's *Political Dictionary*, "The term 'silent majority' refers to a large block of voters that feel marginalized, silenced or underserved by the political system. It's commonly assumed that, if they voted en masse, this 'silent majority' would have an enormous ability to affect the outcome of any given election."

The term was used several times throughout the 1900s but was popularized in 1968 by President Richard Nixon, who was trying to describe the mass of people in the middle who thought that Vice President Hubert Humphrey (the liberal Democratic nominee for president) was an extremist on the left and that George Wallace (the segregationist former governor of Alabama and independent presidential candidate) was an extremist on the right.[8] The silent majority did rally to Nixon that year. He mobilized that massive group and sure enough, he won the presidency in a landslide. This is not about what you think of Nixon. It is about recognizing that "we" collectively have more power than any group in America. "We" can stop the "hijacking" of the narrative in our country. We can stop it in our schools with our young people. We can stop it in the legal system, in the government giveaway system that steals people's agency and self-worth. We can stop it in the erosion of free speech and the seduction of our children by the social media platforms—just to name a few of the many examples we're about to cover.

For our purposes, I'm talking about bringing about a return to traditional values in terms of culture, community, family, and education. And it all requires participation. Because, as I discuss later, silence and passivity too often mean compliance and implicit endorsement.

The other terms you'll see here quite a bit are *cancelled* and *cancel culture*.

Now it gets even more complicated. At its most basic, cancelling is calling someone out for alleged offensive speech and behavior—often on social media in the hopes of silencing them or ensuring that they're held accountable for their words or actions. Depending on your political views, you may feel that "cancel culture" either exists or doesn't exist. And there's a debate as to whether it's a good thing or a bad thing. Some people feel that publicly calling for accountability is an important tool of social justice—a way of combining a lot of voices of people who often don't have power to call out people who they feel have attacked or hurt them.[9] The goal is to deny someone else a following or a platform. But even if someone deserves to be called out, the fear of being cancelled has a chilling effect on all of us. As I alluded to earlier, we now live in an era of "guilt by accusation." No due process, no factual confirmation, just a "gotcha mentality" where lives, families, businesses, and reputations can be destroyed in the court of public opinion, absent facts, data, or a fair opportunity to defend against allegations. True, some bad actors are taken down, but so are a lot of undeserving targets.

People see it happen and can understandably start self-censoring. Those who argue that hearing an opinion with which they disagree can cause emotional stress should also know that there's a body of evidence that shows that *suppressing* an opinion can cause emotional stress. And as I sit here writing, I have two questions. The first is where did this start, or restart? As a country we went decades and decades after the "Red Scare" and McCarthyism of the 1950s—and we recognized that making claims (often baseless) about people and shunning them from public life or getting them fired from their jobs for their opinions had gotten out of control, and was an ugly, ugly chapter in our history. So why has it started again? Perhaps it's because people feel powerless, and the internet gives them the collective power to take down someone they see as powerful, someone whose words or ideas they feel have harmed them.

The second question, and maybe the more important one, is, how can we move from a cancel culture to a healthier "counsel culture"? Or at least a conversation culture. Trust me, it won't be easy, because there are a lot of people out there who want a battle, not a conversation. They want capitulation, not conversion. There are also a lot of people out there who need these conflicts because the conflict gives them meaning, a purpose, and a job. And most of all it gives them attention, *vigilante attention*! They are the self-deputized gotcha police. And they vie to be first on the scene, to crack the biggest case—which usually means catching someone red-handed with the wrong turn of phrase or finding someone who said something wrong (even if it was years and years ago), and then getting as much press as they can out of the perp walk. Many of them in the public eye have had cheap shots taken at them and you may have as well. God forbid peace breaks out, or even just sanity. What would they do then?

What We've Lost

Take a step back and look at where we are as a country. In too many instances we've gotten rid of the most important American trait, self-determination, and replaced it with victimization. We've gotten rid of conversation and replaced it with cancellation. We've gone from courageous to coddled. We've decided to celebrate intent, rather than outcomes. And we're all paying the price for it, spiritually, emotionally, and financially.

We will never, ever whine our way to success (even though social media allows some people to try).

We will never blame our way to fulfillment.

The government will never be able to "entitle" us to self-actualization.

> **In too many instances we've gotten rid of the most important American trait, self-determination, and replaced it with victimization. We've gotten rid of conversation and replaced it with cancellation.**

Government cannot give us that pride of accomplishment that only comes from hard work and observing oneself persevere.

There is no victory in victimhood.

We seem to have forgotten the difference between a "hand up," which we can all use from time to time, and a handout, which starts as a Band-Aid but slowly becomes a crutch, one that if you lean on long enough, you can forget how to walk.

There will never be a sustainable "equality of outcome," no matter how popular the concept. There may never be full equality of opportunity either for that matter.

If you believe in individualism, you must accept individual differences.

We can work on creating equities as a society, but it really is true that you can only "help those who help themselves."

That's where I'm coming from. If you disagree with anything I've said so far, feel free to close the book, hit eject, and move on.

Still with me? Here's my promise.

What I can promise you going forward are facts. You might remember "facts." Facts are what used to be reported before news organizations became propaganda machines trafficking in opinion and selling an agenda.

I can also promise you a formula that works almost every time, if not every time, for creating success in your life, your community, your state, and *our* country.

The formula involves my ten working principles for a healthy society.

And I'm not going to "bury the lede." I'll list them for you right here:

#1: Be Who You Are on Purpose

#2: Focus on Solving Problems Rather Than Winning Arguments

#3: Don't Reward Bad Behavior or Support Conduct You Do Not Value

#4: Measure All Actions Based on Results, and All Thoughts Based on Rationality

#5: Consciously Choose Which Voices in Your Life Deserve the Most Attention

#6: Do Not Stay Silent So Others Can Remain Comfortable

#7: Actively Live and Support a Meritocracy

#8: Identify and Build Your Consequential Knowledge

#9: Work Hard to Understand the Way Others See Things

#10: Treat Yourself and Others with Dignity and Respect

By failing to live by—and live up to—these principles, we have lost so much.

We've lost a sense of perspective. We catastrophize things that are not really catastrophic and, in this process, lose the ability to distinguish between true catastrophes and mere inconveniences or disappointments.

We have lost the tremendous joy and power of gratitude. We have converted charity into entitlement, and thus created donors without love and recipients without gratitude.

We have become intellectually lazy, letting others do our thinking for us. As I'll show in the following pages, that is a deeply dangerous habit. We are not stupid. There are not "versions of the truth." There are certainly different ways of looking at things, but the facts are the facts. Something either happened or it didn't. Things are what they are. People are who they are and they do or don't do what they do or don't do. And all the spin, semantics, and wishing in the world will never change that. Never, ever.

We have abandoned healthy skepticism about what we are told, and in the process set ourselves up to be manipulated and taken advantage of by others. We need to stop being patsies.

We have stopped applying to others the principles we apply to our own children—respect, discipline, individual responsibility, and accountability. Now we reward bad behavior rather than good behavior. The acid test is simply, "Would I do that with respect to my own children?" We need to start applying rules we learned at our mothers' knees.

We have stopped judging actions based on their results. Instead, we judge actions based on intentions or justify them in some other bizarre way. And we've forgotten that age-old wisdom that the road to hell is paved with good intentions.

We have allowed those in power to divide us rather than demanding they unite us.

We have allowed politicians, CEOs, the media, and even—as we'll discuss in the following pages—algorithms to dictate what we do and think. We have ceded our power as citizens and individuals to others. This country was built on the principle that each of us has the individual right to do what we want, to make the choices we want to make, and then to live with the consequences of those choices. We have allowed others to make our choices for us and to create the illusion that they can shield us from the consequences of our conduct. The result is that many of us have gotten in the "comfort zone" of not having to "own our choices" and in the process become the supporting cast rather than *starring in our own lives.* As part of that trade, too many of us have lost the drive to succeed. We have slipped into the tepid sea of collectivist sameness and mediocrity. We need to *star in our own lives.* That means think for ourselves, make our own choices, deal with the consequences of those choices, and celebrate our right to do so.

Too many of us have allowed fear to control our lives and have allowed others to use fear as a means of controlling us, whether it's fear of invoking the Tyranny of the Fringe, or losing our jobs, or fear of actually being attacked. The Bible reminds us, in verse after verse, to "fear not." It is God's directive to us. Research into human nature tells us the number one need in all people is acceptance. The number one fear is rejection. You are not alone in that. We all feel that way.

Some of us have abandoned our faith in the transcendent and in the process have lost the power of belief in a God, as I'll discuss in the "Dangerous Erosion of Faith" chapter. Last year, for the first time, church membership dropped below 50 percent for Americans.[10] We're losing the community and the shared morality that come from organized religion. Sometimes I wonder if too many of us have maybe lost our integrity and moral compass entirely.

Think I'm being a Chicken Little, claiming that the sky is falling? Dr. Phil, c'mon—people still love America. The family unit isn't under attack! People still go to church and get involved in their community. Since I'm guessing you're not a postmodernist, let's take a look at the numbers.

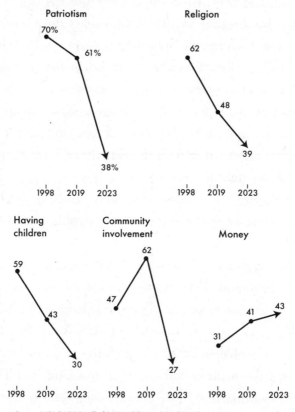

Percent who say these values are "very important" to them

Patriotism

70%
61%
38%

1998 2019 2023

Religion

62
48
39

1998 2019 2023

Having children

59
43
30

1998 2019 2023

Community involvement

62
47
27

1998 2019 2023

Money

41 43
31

1998 2019 2023

Source: WSJ/NORC poll of 1,019 adults conducted March 1–13, 2023; margin of error +/-4.1 pct. pts. Prior data from WSJ/NBC News telephone polls, most recently of 1,000 adults conducted Aug. 10–14, 2019; margin of error +/-3.1 pct. pts.

Even as we become less patriotic, we have come to believe that having the constitutional right to do something makes it the right thing to do. How many times were you told growing up "Just because you *can* doesn't mean you *should*"? I have the constitutional right to burn the American flag, to kneel during our National Anthem, to own a loaded gun and place it on the coffee table with small children running around the house, to say things in anger that are hurtful to ones I love, and to worship the devil. I love that I have rights. I wouldn't sacrifice them for anything. But having the right to do those things doesn't make them the right thing to do.

Again, we have forgotten the most important thing for success in our own lives—our individual selves. We have forgotten that each of us is the captain of our own fate, the master of our own soul. We have taken handouts, material and intellectual, from others, and in the process have become beholden to them. My friend Chase Hughes, whom you'll meet a little later, says that when a problem becomes so large, there's a tendency to become apathetic. It's almost like we start to say, "I can't deal with this, so I'm not even going to try." He calls it "societally programmed apathy."

But for me, it all comes back to this: having some sense of control over the outcome of your life as an individual is extremely important to having the courage to redefine the narrative of today's America as a country.

It is the firm footing on which you can dig in and stand up against ideological bullies, fearmongers, media, and technology companies—anyone using emotional extortion to shape, manipulate, use, or silence you. So, before you read on, resolve to do away with the apathy. You can deal with this. And you're about to.

POLL RESPONSE

How concerned are you that "fringe groups" are trying to hijack and displace core values, scientific findings, and an unbiased view of history in America?

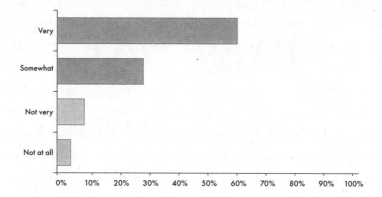

Again, ask yourself how you fit in to this survey response. Remember there's not a right or wrong answer. You're not wrong if you're part of that or not part of it. I just want you to know where you stand in comparison to a national survey comprised of people, many of whom are Dr. Phil viewers, but not all. This will all come together when you've answered all of the questions throughout this book.

PART ONE

America's Daily Focus
Has Changed

I've seen this storm brewing for some time.

Because of my platform, I've had a chance to be the canary in the cultural coal mine.

For years, challenges that guests brought to us have focused mostly on human functioning—how to live better lives.

But in recent years, instead of categories of questions that could be defined as dealing with the psychology of individuals, relationships, and families, we began to notice additional concerns about broader, more socially oriented issues. We started hearing about these additional concerns and strong anxieties about what was happening in our viewers' *collective* experiences. What was happening culturally in their communities, places of employment, churches, their children's elementary and secondary schools, their online communities, and what they were being bombarded with by the media. It was different topics and a different tone, marked by "unrest" and trepidation. I sensed an overlay of mental and emotional disorientation, and even fear.

The disorientation was characterized by recurring statements like:

What's going on?

Things seem to be so out of control, I wonder if we are going to be okay.

I'm feeling "judged" about my beliefs even in *my own home*.

I'm afraid to even open my mouth, afraid I don't know the right "words of the week"! I've seen people get labeled "hater" so fast at my job, it was frightening.

Am I supposed to feel like a "racist" just because I'm white? I keep getting messages that I'm supposed to feel guilty, but I don't know what I'm supposed to stop doing!

What do I tell my kids about going to school when shootings are plastered all over the news? I can't honestly tell them, "It will be okay."

My son is transgender and I have absolutely no idea, not one clue, what to say or do to help him? Do I support him? Do I get him counseling and if so *for what*? Does this mean he is gay? I'm lost but he is getting picked on, bullied, and mocked. He said he has been using a girl's name at school for the last three months! What is he talking about? HELP?

I'm watching employees, security guards, and even cops watch thieves empty shelves in our drugstore and do nothing. What am I missing? Why *am I* paying?

Why don't you white people get it? I'm Black and I don't have half a chance. I can't even rent an apartment near my job. They won't even *show* me a condo I'm willing to pay asking price for. What do I do with this anger? Nobody gets it.

How are our kids buying drugs on social media? I thought that was all about music and funny videos?

We both work. We are scared to death the "speech police" are going to cancel one or both of us because we chose the wrong word or gave the wrong opinion. We're not up to speed on all of this, and we've got other things to worry about. Gas by our house is so expensive we can't afford to even eat lunch. If one of us gets fired, we are so screwed. The stress is killing us and we weren't getting along that great to begin with.

I'm a single mom with two kids in college so they can get better jobs. All they seem to focus on is ideas about "the system." My daughter said I was a "capitalist"! She is supposed to be studying business management! Why am I working two jobs?

As I write this, there have been over four hundred mass shootings in 2023. Have we just gone crazy? I'm afraid to go out, and if I bring it up half the people treat me like I'm the one with a problem! Help!

Since when did we rewrite biology? I'm so confused and said so in the cafeteria at work and now I've been written up for asking a question.

I could erase every one of those statements (all closely paraphrased) and replace them with a dozen others and, taken as a whole, they would convey the same overall feeling of emotional disorientation, frustration, anger, fear, and intimidation.

If I had to characterize them broadly, they'd fall under the heading of "What the hell is going on in this country?"

These questions aren't just about "functioning"—which is how I describe the questions that are about the psychology of individuals.

They're about *survival*. Economic, professional, and reputational survival. And even *actual survival*. Literal survival—from school shootings and violence. And when you read between the lines, the people writing me are clearly concerned about our very survival as a nation as the family-based country we all know.

They all seem to share concerns about this "cancel culture" where if you disagree with the wrong person or you say the wrong word, somebody jumps up and points the accusatory finger and yells, "Hate speech!" So many people—good, hardworking people with love in their hearts—seem to be living under this Tyranny of the Fringe I've been writing about already. Notice I didn't say "tyranny of the minority," because I don't think there are even enough of these "cultural disruptors" to even be described as a minority.

This is a very small group of people who live, think, and behave on the outermost fringes, on both ends of the spectrum.

This is not about a bunch of fuddy-duddys being resistant to societal change either. I love change, I embrace change. We all need to challenge ourselves to get out of our "comfort zones" from time to time and evolve and grow.

But that doesn't mean we find the most bizarre, unsupported, nonscientific ideology we can, embrace it, and send a message to the world: *Suspend critical thinking! Ignore centuries of science. The loudmouth over there has it right!*

We often say (at least I hope we often say) that America is a great country.

But we don't often remind ourselves of why it is a great country.

This country got to the place of being the example to which the world aspires through hard work by its citizens, intellectual honesty, unified effort, freedom of thought, speech, and religion, respect for our fellow man, and the rule of law.

This book is the result of a decision I have made: that I will not and, in fact, cannot continue to ignore the psychological reality, the cultural certainty, that if we continue down the path we are on, a path that says we can stop thinking rationally, reward intentions rather than results, allow the loudest voices to drown out everything else, dole out rewards independent of effort, ignore legitimate, properly arrived-at, replicated scientific findings just because we may not like them, attack rather than have compassion for our fellow man, fail to have a sense of pride in America, and care more about winning arguments than solving problems—we are going to see this great country continue to slide down the scale of excellence.

Truly, I mean that. You can draw a straight line from those destructive impulses to the fact that kids aren't getting the education they need, businesses aren't getting the employees they need, people aren't living the lives they deserve, and America is losing our understanding of the power of self-determination. Bad attitudes, bad outcomes.

Sure, staying silent may allow others to remain comfortable. Heck, it might allow me to remain comfortable. Rest assured I know I will be targeted and attacked for giving voice to what I am seeing. But there's no comfort in knowing that we are tearing up the greatest country in the world, and we're doing it because a small number of disconnected people want to complain, spread discontent, and push agendas many of which have no foundation whatsoever. How is that working for us? Seriously, is there any theory under which that makes sense? You can never let the tail wag the dog.

Perhaps you are thinking, "Whoa! Hold on there, Doc, it can't be that bad. Aren't you being a bit dramatic? I'm still living my life, watching television, following my favorite sports team, listening to music, walking my dog, doing everyday stuff. How bad can it be?"

The answer is, bad.

> **If you don't feel the urgency, it's only because you're like the proverbial frog in the pot of water that's being turned up to a boil. Even if you don't feel it, it's coming for you.**

If you don't feel the urgency, it's only because you're like the proverbial frog in the pot of water that's being turned up to a boil. Even if you don't feel it, it's coming for you. I wish I was being overly dramatic, but I'm not, not by a long shot.

Think about it another way: Imagine you're enjoying a nice walk along a country road, earphones in, listening to music. I'm walking toward you. I can see what you can't see: there's a giant eighteen-wheeler careening out of control coming up on you, headed straight for you. You would definitely want me to tell you! You would want me to shout out an unmistakable warning to alert you to the immediate, imminent danger. You'd want me to run to you and heave you out of harm's way. To do any less would be grossly negligent. That's the analogy I have in my head as I am writing this and raising this alarm.

POLL RESPONSE

Looking back at the past year, how often did you find yourself worrying about an issue of basic survival, such as personal safety or the ability to provide for yourself and your family?

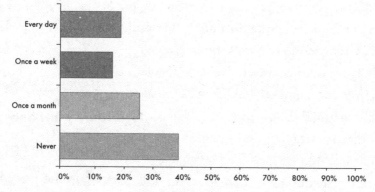

According to the responses, some of you see this as a big problem. Some of you don't think it's a problem at all. Again, no right or wrong answer. You'll read more about that as we move along.

CHAPTER 2

Think Freely, Speak Freely

POLL QUESTION

Is there a difference between getting your "feelings hurt" by words and being "injured" by someone saying something offensive to you?

- ☐ No difference
- ☐ Not much difference
- ☐ Some difference
- ☐ No similarity

Words Can Hurt

Now, I'm going to say something that might surprise you, something you might not expect to hear "from a buck up, suck up" character like me: words can hurt.

Now, before you accuse me of going full snowflake, or contradicting what I have written earlier, let me add some context, starting with an experiment.

I want you to imagine the coldest, freshest dill pickle you can imagine. Can you smell it, the garlic and dill? Can you taste that vinegary, acidic brine on your tongue?

I'd put the contents of my wallet on the fact that you're salivating right now.

That's because the thoughts we have, the words we speak and hear, do have physiological correlates.

A study conducted in 2019 found that when patients were shown words that were linked with pain (like *excruciating*), they found the procedure more painful than patients who were shown words that weren't linked with pain.[1]

And of course, I've spoken to countless patients for whom prolonged verbal abuse—verbal, not physical abuse—led to anxiety and chronic pain, and the science backs this up.[2]

Words matter.

Words have an impact.

I don't deny it. I'm saying let's not catastrophize things that aren't catastrophic.

And let's be especially cognizant of what we say to ourselves. We've just talked about how words that we see or that others say to us can affect us. But those are no match for the power of our "internal dialogue." Keeping that dialogue neutral to positive is important for a whole host of reasons. Two of the most important ones are:

We tend to believe what we tell ourselves. So, if you are being negative, if you are being critical and doubting your ability to succeed or overcome a challenge, you are likely to believe yourself and live *down* to your expectations.

Just as important is the need to recognize that people typically speak at a pace of about 120 words per minute but think at about 1,200–1,400 words per minute! This is incredibly important because if someone—a bully or critic perhaps—says something designed to undermine your confidence, they may say it to or about you one time. But if you internalize and start running it through your head over and over, you are doing it at 10X speed!

And for a lot of reasons, our internal dialogue has a negative bias. It tends to believe and repeat the negative stories.

Some of you may have seen the Dove "real beauty" films. In one film, a series of women are the subject of two portraits drawn by an FBI-trained forensic artist. The catch is, he doesn't look at the women—he draws off of two different descriptions. The first portrait is the woman describing herself. They tend to say things like "my lips are too thin" or "my chin is too big" or "I have wrinkles around my eyes."

The second portrait is a stranger describing the same woman. And you tend to hear things like "she has a nice smile" and "she has nice cheekbones."

The women are then shown the two portraits, and they see the difference between how they see themselves, and how others see them. When each woman is shown the difference between how she sees herself and how a stranger sees her, she's shocked, because she sees how unkind she's being to herself. I would argue she sees how cruel her internal dialogue can be—as cruel as any bully.

And I've seen it in my own work.

Sometimes I'll ask a guest, "Tell me what you really do not like about yourself." They can talk for thirty minutes, barely taking a breath: "I'm lazy, I'm an addict, I'm worthless . . ."

Then I'll say, "Okay, I got it, but I don't care how flat you make a pancake, it's still got two sides. So now tell me five *good* things about you." Often they just sit there and stare at the floor for the longest time. It's as though they're looking for a lost contact lens. And then they'll just burst into tears because they can't think of a single thing or, if they can, they can't bring themselves to say it out loud.

Yes, words can hurt.

And our minds are tricky places.

Because in some cases, words can also help. For some of us, when we redirect our minds to focus on the positives, when we affirm our positive traits, we activate the reward centers in the brain.[3] Some researchers report that if you have an optimistic outlook, a positive mindset, it can increase your productivity by over 30 percent. I don't know about you, but I can sure use the extra percentage points!

But for people with low self-esteem to begin with, positive, affirming self-talk actually makes you feel more negatively about yourself—because you don't believe the positive words.[4]

Because of this, the most important thing we can do is build our resilience to hurtful words, because we can't avoid them. They're always going to exist in our internal dialogue. And that's why the attempt to avoid words that might hurt is so misguided.

Trigger Warning

To ease you into that greater resilience, I need to offer a trigger warning. The trigger warning is this: trigger warnings have become the most unadulterated load of BS you may ever come across. At best, they're ineffective. At worst, the warnings themselves are as traumatic as any content that they could ever warn you about. And the very fact of their existence reflects two seriously unhealthy trends that are being pushed so hard by some factions that it is beyond ridiculous.

If you've never personally come across the term *trigger warning* or an actual trigger warning before, here's what they are: they are announcements that provide readers of a book, viewers of a show or movie, or listeners of a lecture that something they're about to see could be disturbing and trigger a strong emotional response.

The question I have been turning over in my mind as I watch the continued proliferation of these trigger warnings is: Are the supposedly enlightened individuals, factions, and organizations peddling this wholly dysfunctional concept knowingly misguiding everyone (which would make them toxic saboteurs)? Or are they just so lazy or arrogant that they haven't bothered to investigate the available research to see if what they are advocating is actually helpful or hurtful?

That is my problem with so much of their well-publicized agenda—it's supported by ideology rather than evidence. And policies and decisions based on ideology rather than evidence tend not to work.

We see ideology over evidence in the conduct of the woke prosecutors and judges who think they are revolutionizing jurisprudence by "compassionately" releasing repeat offenders back on the street because they say we incarcerate too many citizens. That may be, but evidence shows that putting violent perpetrators back in the public sphere among an innocent and unsuspecting public is not working as a solution. Ideology over evidence can also be seen in the college professors who are sabotaging young men by convincing them that aggression in the business world is somehow unbecoming and unenlightened, and in the untrained school board members sexualizing young children without a clue—I mean *no clue*—about developmental biology or the long-term ramifications of their actions just so they can feel, what? Cutting-edge? Forward-thinking?

It's easy to enact your ideology when you don't have to be around for the crash, when you have no accountability down the road, when you don't have to worry about the ever-growing pile of evidence that the outcome ain't what you expected.

This is the same mindset that leads someone to defend the shoplifters who are robbing stores blind. These shoplifters justify theft because they believe they deserve a certain standard of living in pursuit of equality of outcome. I wonder how their defenders would feel if it was their house being robbed from or their vehicle being carjacked. It is always easier to support in the abstract, but if you walk around all day preaching ideology, at some point evidence is going to sneak up and punch you in the face. I could go on (and will) in the pages that follow, but all of these issues share the premise that no one is ever accountable, everyone is the victim of something, science doesn't matter, and everyone is entitled to be "taken care of."

Trigger warnings are a great example of a misguided ideological agenda. But the evidence is clear: their implications are so much more far-reaching than meets the eye. And by the way, the problems with trigger warnings are *knowable* if someone is interested in the facts rather than "virtue signaling." It is terrible to mess up someone's life just to make yourself look "with it."

The first trend is that this scientifically unsupported concept conditions people to believe that they deserve—in fact are entitled to—protection from life itself, from words, images, and ideas just because those exposures might stress them or even distress them.

.They wish to be "warned" so they can "turtle up" and hide from the content, rather than develop the necessary resilience to content that can be upsetting. It conditions them to think that avoidance is healthy and possible when in fact these experiences are unequivocally unavoidable. This mindset encourages people to adopt an extremely limiting, low-self-esteem image in which they have little or no confidence to face the demands of life.

Second, it robs those who lean on or hide behind trigger warnings of the opportunity to master their environment by overcoming obstacles, completing demanding tasks, or achieving difficult goals. A critical part of life and development is gone because people who don't know what they are doing wish life to be nothing but smooth sailing. As a result, they start trying to get other people to join their fantasyland concept and to pretend right along with them. Such a fanciful attitude, adopted by so many, comes at a very high cost: a significant portion of an entire generation groomed to hide from the demands of life rather than get competent, get tough, and get confident in their ability to handle the demands of life.

Some colleges even have "safe rooms" for students who feel "triggered" or fear they may be because of life's traumas, like an election turning out differently than they had hoped, or a speaker or professor that dared to disagree with or challenge them! I am totally serious and, again, this would be a good place to fact-check me. Research "college safe rooms, stress, coloring books, puppies." Yes, you read that right, "coloring books and puppies." What better preparation for a competitive world.

The term *trigger warning* first started appearing in the early 2000s, and it seems that it was designed to protect people who were at risk of experiencing post-traumatic stress disorder (PTSD). For example, if you had experienced child abuse, a warning would let you know that you were about to be exposed to the topic of child abuse in some forum. Warnings like this may have made sense in isolated cases of severe, or yet-to-be-treated or -processed PTSD—especially where violent assault or rape were still very raw emotionally. Maybe? The question would then become whether you can really identify what actually triggers a reaction by an affected individual. Sometimes it is not a logical cue or reminder.

But, like almost everything today, a coddled generation got ahold of trigger warnings and were soon requesting them everywhere and for everything, not just recent, raw victims of violent crimes or events.

They became disconnected from things that could actually trigger PTSD or even a transient reaction to a prior bad experience, and became a sort of moral catch-all. They became a tool and rallying cry for those wishing to "virtue signal" that they are somehow "supersensitive" and dialed into the plight of the vulnerable. And for a coddled generation, they became a constant request, and an admission that they were comfortable in the role of the delicate victim. Both groups now hide behind the demand for warnings in a ridiculously broad number of categories.

A prime example occurred at Oberlin College in 2014, when administrators advised faculty members to "understand triggers, avoid unnecessary triggers, and provide trigger warnings" because something that "recalls a traumatic event to an individual" would "disrupt a student's learning and may make some students feel unsafe in your classroom."[5]

As a result, we ended up with the surreal example in which Oberlin noted, "Chinua Achebe's *Things Fall Apart* . . . may trigger readers who have experienced racism, colonialism, religious persecution, violence, suicide, and more."[6]

I mean, you might as well have a trigger warning that says, "You're about to read a story about people. Bad things happen to people. Especially because there aren't many books where only good things happen to people." The list of potential triggers is endless, of course. And that's the problem. At least Oberlin saw the light and dropped the policy.

But the virus had already escaped the lab. By 2016, a survey found that half of college and university teachers had used trigger warnings in their teaching. And we started seeing them pop up everywhere.

We now see demands online and in the classroom for subject matters as wide-ranging as divorce, patriarchy, misogyny, diets, the death penalty, calories being indicated on food packaging, terrorism, drug consumption, certain ideological positions, "painful" political or electoral outcomes, drug use, drunk driving, weight, racism, gun violence, homophobia, slavery, victim-blaming, body-shaming, abuse, child abuse, cutting, suicide, surgery, plane crashes, corpses, skulls, skeletons, needles, discussion of "isms," stuttering, slurs, kidnapping, dental trauma, sexual activity (even consensual), death, spiders, insects, snakes, vomit, pregnancy, childbirth, blood, and mental illness, just to name a few.

The Globe Theatre in London offered a trigger warning for Shakespeare's *Romeo and Juliet*. The triggers? Upsetting themes including suicide and drug use. Not only was that probably the world's most unnecessary trigger warning, it's also a spoiler alert!

One philosophy professor at Cornell University justified the use of trigger warnings by saying, "Exposing students to triggering material without warning seems more akin to occasionally throwing a spider at an arachnophobe."[7]

And of course, you don't throw spiders at people who are terrified of them. But if you're a law student who signs up for a class on rape law, and you—God forbid—have been raped, you know what you've signed up for. You're not throwing a spider at an arachnophobe. The arachnophobe has chosen to go into a room where they know there will be pictures of spiders.

The reason I get particularly exercised about seeing these trigger warnings in college courses is that college is the place to, wait for it . . . learn! Get exposed to what you *are not* comfortable with. Art, literature, philosophy, science. It is the opportunity and the setting to explore new ideas, expand knowledge, interrogate power, confront difficult truths, and learn how to make an argument and to read a text. I admit college isn't meant to be "therapy." It isn't exactly the real world either, but it should approximate the real world more than your mother's lap! It is, hopefully, a space to be challenged, tested, frustrated, even big-time upset. Sure, there are some times and places where you should meet someone exactly where they are. But not in a place that is dedicated to expanding horizons. Students should accept the challenge of exploring their own beliefs and engaging in disagreement.

Trigger warnings do not encourage that discourse or, for that matter, any discourse. Trigger warnings deflect, avoid, and in yet another setting cheat the student out of observing themselves overcome uncomfortable feelings, or learn how to cope with stress and distress. What's more, this is not reflective of the real world. In the real world, every upsetting—even emotionally devastating—piece of information and content, activity, challenge, experience, or conflict will most definitely not come with a trigger warning because life is unpredictable. You can't hit pause and pop up a warning!

If college is meant to prepare the student for the next level of life, then colleges are cheating their students miserably by coddling them with these trigger warnings.

Once again, trauma has been defined down. Students are allowed to hide behind their "triggers," and a trigger can be as simple as disliking or being mildly uncomfortable with some content. We see a similar impulse in people who self-victimize online. Sometimes it seems like these people are fighting over who can be the most traumatized rather than devoting their energy toward seeking health.

Think about it this way: we lived for centuries without trigger warnings and got by just fine.

Now, you might also say we lived a long time without antibiotics. But we were sure happy when in 1909 German physician Paul Ehrlich discovered arsphenamine for treating syphilis, and nineteen long years later in 1928 when Alexander Fleming discovered penicillin.

True, but those medicines represented real progress supported by irrefutable science and real-world results—results that saved millions of lives.

Not so with trigger warnings. No science to be found here. No lives saved or improved either. On the contrary, trigger warnings fly in the face of the actual science, which is that it's almost impossible to avoid that which you fear, so the best course is to prepare yourself to be exposed to it. This is "exposure therapy," and it is what is called an "evidence-based therapy," meaning that it does work.

There is an impressive body of evidence demonstrating that people in general and certainly those experiencing varying levels of fear and anxiety can be helped by exposure rather than avoidance of stimuli from which the trigger warnings seek to protect them.

Dialectical behavioral therapy (DBT) is another evidenced-based therapy that, like exposure therapy, works on modifying internal dialogue. Much like cognitive behavior therapy (CBT), these approaches help individuals learn to cope with and manage stress and problems in life rather than avoid or hide from them.

DBT helps people develop healthy ways to cope with demands and control their emotions, rather than letting their emotions control them.

CBT, DBT, and exposure therapy are all tried and proven techniques; far superior to living a life avoiding stimuli, events, and circumstances that might upset you.

Knowing how to cope widens your world; it allows for freedom and power. Freedom from fear. Power to navigate the world with resilience. Allowing people to hide behind trigger warnings denies them the opportunity to develop resilience.

By now, I'm sure you realize that my approach to psychology is that you cannot avoid the things in this world you fear. It's just not possible. And it's a recipe for retaining that fear for life.

If you almost drown once when you're young, you can't avoid water for the rest of your life. You have to learn to wade into the water. And then put your head underwater. And then swim. That's basically what exposure therapy is. You have to become resilient to that which you fear.

Trigger warnings simply don't work.

Not only do trigger warnings promote a culture of avoidance and oversensitivity; by warning individuals in advance about potentially upsetting content, trigger warnings prevent people from engaging with challenging or uncomfortable material and instead reinforce the belief that they are fragile and in need of protection.

Furthermore, many studies suggest that trigger warnings are not effective at treating trauma or reducing distress, and that they may even be detrimental to mental health by preventing individuals from confronting and processing their emotions.

Another thing to consider: Even people who have experienced trauma are rarely "triggered" by the obvious thing you think might trigger them. A victim of rape, for example, might not be triggered by a rape scene in a movie, but by the ticking of a clock that sounds similar to the one she heard at the time. Sometimes for a victim of

> **Knowing how to cope widens your world; it allows for freedom and power. Freedom from fear. Power to navigate the world with resilience.**

trauma, it's a certain smell or scent that will bring them back. The mind is a complicated place.

But what we do know is that several studies have shown that trigger warnings are worse than no warning at all. One study conducted at Harvard surveyed people who said that they believe that words can cause harm. Among that group of people, the trigger warning about what they were about to read caused more anxiety than the passage itself.

They've become a way to "coddle" students (we'll discuss coddling in a bit) and keep them from having to engage with ideas that might challenge their beliefs, to remind you that you might once have been a victim of something, and make victimization a key part of your identity (we'll discuss that you're not a victim in a bit), and to impose someone else's view of what's harmful in your life (and we're going to discuss *you* determining what you want in your own life *a lot*).

Finally, trigger warnings infringe on academic freedom and hinder the discussion and exploration of complex issues in the classroom by limiting the range of material that can be covered.

But Dr. Phil, why are you so worked up about a trigger warning? About a couple of words at the beginning of a class or a play or a movie?

Because trigger warnings are a symptom of a much larger problem.

Let me explain it the best way I know how.

I'm a licensed pilot and have been since my teens. I have several thousand hours of pilot-in-command time under my belt. The way you get that many hours without flying being your full-time career is to fly a lot of slow airplanes—the slower you go, the longer it takes to get anywhere!

When I was learning, my flight instructor told me that rough air was a fact of flying, and he knew I would be stubborn about my "go-no, go" decisions. Meaning, he knew that I would have a bias toward "go," so he'd better train me very well to fly safely with turbulence.

My older sister, Deana, also took flying lessons from the same instructor. To say she did not like turbulence is to put it mildly. She looked at the wind the way a long-tailed cat looks at a room full of rocking chairs—nervously.

But Deana, I'm proud to say, was committed, and she managed to get her private pilot's license. But when she flew, she seldom got out of sight of the airport, flew with a giant stuffed Snoopy dog in the passenger seat, and only went out on days when it was "severe clear" and millpond calm—days when you could drop a feather and have it float straight down between your feet.

There were a lot of days she just could not fly. If the flag was flying, Deana was not. If the flag was hanging limp by the pole, off she went!

I was taught to cope with the wind, even winds so strong that you had to lean into them to walk. Which meant that I felt perfectly confident flying most days.

One day, I was doing an instrument training flight with my instructor and Deana decided to hop in the back for fun. We had been up about an hour and were crossing over the Red River, from Oklahoma to Texas. We were flying below a cloud deck at night when, in a freakish turn of bad luck, we got sucked up into a thunderstorm that was "hiding" in the overcast, evening clouds.

We went from smooth to really, really rough air in a matter of seconds.

We got rattled around pretty good. Up front, the Klaxon bleat of the stall warning was going off. The sound of the rain hammering the plane was deafening. I think at one point we were actually inverted. It was so violent that to have resisted the up- and downdrafts could well have snapped the wings off the airplane. But by the grace of God and staying "hooked up to it" we got through it and got back on the ground, a little green around the gills but not significantly worse for the wear. (A saying among pilots is that you should always fly with a magnetic compass, a cat, and a duck: the duck won't fly in bad weather, the cat always lands on its feet, and the compass will get you home.)

My and my instructor's first thought was to walk around the plane and check for structural damage. We really thought that we might find that some of the rivets holding the outer skin on the plane had popped loose. We wanted to be sure we weren't missing any parts—at least not any parts we needed. Deana, on the other hand, was white as a sheet. She crawled out on the wing of that plane like a shipwrecked sailor crawling up on a beach.

She backed herself down onto the ground, crying—sobbing really.

She steadied herself and I put my hand on her shoulder in hopes of calming her.

"Don't you touch me! Don't you ever talk to me again, either one of you!"

Then she cussed me out, in a way that would have made that shipwrecked sailor I alluded to earlier blush!

Sadly, Deana passed away recently, and I miss her terribly.

We had a lot of good memories together—before and after that flight.

But in the decades after that night, she never piloted a small plane again.

I hated that for her. I talked to her about it, but it was nonnegotiable.

I flew the next afternoon.

I did have weather radar installed on that and every airplane I've ever owned since that night so I could "see" what can't be seen. But I definitely kept flying.

I attribute her reaction purely to the fact that she had no preparation and no expectation of experiencing any kind of turbulence, certainly not anything like what we went through.

I truly believe it is not what happens in life that causes us to be upset.

It's the *violations of what we expect to happen* in life that causes us to be upset.

If you expect A and you get A, no problem.

But if you expect A and you get B, now you may have a problem.

If you expect A and you get Z, you will likely have a *big* problem.

Trigger warnings are just another way that we're teaching people to live their lives where the feather floats down between their feet. Only ever expect A and run away or shut your eyes so you never even have to consider dealing with B or S or even Z.

Remember, your reaction to life isn't about what happens. It's about what you expect to happen and the story you *tell yourself* about what happens.

When you don't get A and you tell yourself something must be seriously wrong, it could lead to real panic.

Effective therapies work at getting you to tell a better story to yourself.

For example, exposure therapy is about gaining power over the story by desensitizing yourself.

Dialectical behavior therapy works with people to talk through their experiences as a way of understanding and accepting reality.

Both therapies recognize that sheltering and shielding people from reality is not a solution.

If you expect turbulence and you have to fly through it, you can deal with it.

If you expect financial stress and you experience it, you can weather it.

If you expect marital trouble and you encounter it, you can work through it.

If you teach your child to expect some bullying, exclusion, and name-calling, they'll be able to handle it.

But today, rather than preparing people to deal with reality, we're creating a fiction that they can avoid reality, but, at some point or another, reality will catch up with them.

We see the benefits of "exposure" in other areas of medicine too. Doctors have come to realize that exposure to germs makes you healthier in the long run—and that overdoing cleanliness and scrubbing every surface with antiseptic wipes can lead to allergies and asthma.[8]

The same goes for exposure to challenges in life. Resilience matters, and resilience comes from experiencing adversity.

You can't legislate away stress, challenges, and obstacles. There are always issues people are going to have to deal with. Wishing that something was or wasn't the case works until you walk out in the real world; then you realize the truth of the old saying: wish in one hand and spit in the other, and see which one fills up first.

Life is going to spit at you. Life is going to violate your hopes and expectations. How you react to that is what defines you.

Sheltering and shielding does nothing to prepare children for life.

We need to teach people to cope, not avoid. Persevere, not be protected.

We want people to be able to fly in all conditions every day.

And trigger warnings won't protect you. Learning to navigate turbulence will.

In talking about trigger warnings, I quoted the Cornell professor for a reason. That's because this ridiculousness came home to roost there recently. Students passed a resolution that called on the university to require faculty to provide trigger warnings about traumatic content that could be presented in class, "including but not limited to: sexual assault, domestic violence, self-harm, suicide, child abuse, racial hate crimes, transphobic violence, homophobic harassment, xenophobia." What's more, the resolution said that students who chose to opt out of exposure wouldn't be penalized.[9]

The university responded, "We cannot accept this resolution, as the actions it recommends would infringe on our core commitment to academic freedom and freedom of inquiry."

I breathed a sigh of relief when I saw that.

Maybe, just maybe, the pendulum is starting to swing back.

And if an ivory-tower Ivy League school can stand up to this nonsense, you can too.

POLL RESPONSE

Is there a difference between getting your "feelings hurt" by words and being "injured" by someone saying something offensive to you?

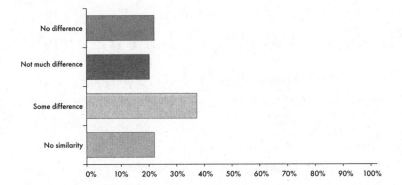

This question, in retrospect may have been a little nuanced, and I wrote it already knowing a lot about some of the differences. The distinction was drawing a line between emotional impact and physical, medical impact. So, if you want to think through that again after reading this chapter and reconsider your answer, you can. That will take on some significance as we move forward.

CHAPTER 3

"Inclusive Language" Isn't Inclusive, and It's Barely Language

---

POLL QUESTION

In the last year, have you struggled to remember the "right" word you're supposed to use to describe someone or something in a way you consider to be sensitive, in a situation or a conversation that might be sensitive?

- ☐ Always
- ☐ Very Often
- ☐ Sometimes
- ☐ Never

Not only are we allowing these bullies to rob us of our right to our free expression, but we're allowing these same fringe factions, activists, and ideologues to actually rewrite history and eradicate individual words by the basketful.

I feel like our glossary is changing so quickly that keeping up has become a full-time job. It's absurd. And if you fail to keep up, woe unto you. You could get labeled with the suffix *-phobic*.

I live my life in public, and there are people "grading my paper" every single day. And every day, I wonder when, despite my best intentions, I'm going to "step in it" word-wise. (More realistically, how often!) And when you or I do, as is inevitable since we don't always have time to keep up with the glossary of the week for every group, it won't matter if it was a misspeak, an honest, unintended mistake of ignorance. It won't matter what was in your heart or how you really feel. What will matter is "THEY GOTCHA! THEY GOT ONE!" They will alert the press, call your employer, threaten to boycott any business affiliated with you or your company. This is "cancel culture," not "counsel culture." There is no interest in talking or educating, because you are a prop! You are no longer a person (if you ever were); you are a hater, a means to get publicity about how victimized the group is. Never mind that you are anything but a hater. You become grist for the publicity mill.

Heaven forbid you refer to the room you sleep in as the "master bedroom" instead of the "primary bedroom"—you must be a racist, slave-owning plantation owner at heart.[1]

Except you're not allowed to say "slave"—the correct term now is "enslaved person." Look, I'm not saying there's not a good point here. Masters did terrible things, and to call someone a slave takes away their humanity. But using the wrong term ain't the same as endorsing where it came from.

Some of these "rules" go way too far. In fact they lead people into picking the wrong battles. If I am going to seriously fight racism in America, and that is a battle worth fighting, it won't focus on how someone refers to their bedroom. They aren't masters and didn't own slaves.

Heck, you're not even supposed to say "American," according to Stanford University's inclusive language guide.[2] And why not? Because saying "American" implies "that the U.S. is the most important country in the Americas." And by the way, if you're interested in attending the schools that have become training academies for the language police, don't go looking for the *admissions office*. Because "admissions" means that someone might have to be "rejected." Look for, and I kid you not, the "office of enrollment management."

Reading all of the words you can't say makes me want to say some things you *really* can't say.

Consider the University of Washington's Inclusive Language Guide.

In this guide, the university's Information Technology department says they are "involved in activities to replace racist, sexist, ageist, ableist, homophobic or otherwise non-inclusive language scattered throughout materials and resources in the software and information technology fields."[3]

This is a fine goal—using language that makes people feel included.

But then look at some of the words that they flag.

Like a "brown bag" lunch, which you shouldn't say because certain African American sororities and fraternities used brown lunch bags to judge skin color. So, to invite someone to a brown bag lunch "surfaces an ugly period of American history that can alienate and offend people." Of course, maybe, just maybe, I'm just simply bringing my lunch in an actual bag that is brown, and am saying if we meet up, you should too. Honestly does anyone actually believe we will become a better country if Bob doesn't say to Jeff, "Hey, let's just brown-bag it tomorrow in the park at twelve thirty and throw the Frisbee around instead of sitting in a cafeteria somewhere"?

We're not supposed to say "native or non-native" speaker anymore, because "English is not the native language of the land occupied by the United States of America."

Or "Sherpa," "ninja," or "guru," which you shouldn't say because even though anytime I use them, you can bet it's in the form of a compliment to an expert or guide, I'm told "these words are culturally appropriative." No kidding. *Words* are culturally appropriative! We take them from everywhere.

Again, believe it or not, I don't want to offend anyone.

I *want* to use language that respects the people I'm talking to, and about. But there are literally hundreds of common words on these lists, and I guarantee you that I'll run afoul of one of them at some point. (Can I say afoul? Is it offensive to chickens? It's not? Good, I really ducked one there. Wait, is that offensive to ducks?)

I don't want to be attacked as a racist or phobic.

Now the Associated Press has entered the fray. They're the group of reporters whose "stylebook" sends a signal of what language Americans should be using. So, you can imagine my reaction when they announced, "We recommend avoiding general and often dehumanizing 'the' labels such as *the* poor, *the* mentally ill, *the* French, *the* disabled, *the* college educated." Hold on a second. Has anyone ever felt *insulted* by being called "the college educated"?

Do the French feel insulted by being called "the French"? Apparently not, because the French (oops) embassy in the United States joked that it now had to change its name to the "Embassy of Frenchness." France's spokesperson later said, "We just wondered what the alternative to 'the French' would be."[4] I have never agreed with a French government official more.

The attempt to change our language to make it more inclusive is doing just the opposite. I grew up in Texas and Oklahoma (and a lot of other places). A lot of the people I know here who came from Mexico or Central or South America will either describe themselves with the country they or their family came from (Mexican American, Colombian American, and so on), or, more generally, they'll call themselves Latino, Latina, or Hispanic. I've never heard a single person call themselves Latinx. Latinx is supposed to be a gender-neutral way of saying Latina or Latino, because in Spanish, like lots of languages, nouns ending with an *o* are male, and words ending with an *a* are female. So, I suppose in some way, it makes sense to try to find a gender-neutral word, until you realize it makes no sense at all. A poll done of people of Latin American descent showed that 76 percent had never even heard the term *Latinx*. Only 3 percent use it.[5] Another poll found that 40 percent of Latinos found the word *offensive*.[6] And here's why—it erases the way things work in another language, and replaces it with an English word, and not just any English word, but an English word that seems to be used only by overly woke white liberals and intellectuals. It's the opposite of sensitive. The opposite of inclusive. It's just ridiculous.

And by the way, the exact same thing is true for the term *BIPOC*, which, if you haven't yet been indoctrinated, stands for Black, Indigenous, and People of Color.[7] Sounds pretty inclusive, except white Democrats like the term twice as much as *actual* people of color.[8] And Asians and Latinos aren't sure whether they're considered people of color. And a significant number of people misinterpret it to mean *bisexual* people of color, which it's not intended to mean. So, this attempt to be inclusive does the opposite; it confuses and confounds.

And the ridiculousness doesn't end there. *Homeless* is now a no-no word. Suggested alternatives are *houseless* (I guess a house is not a home), *unhoused*, or "people experiencing homelessness" (it's about the people, not the houses).[9] How about we spend less time developing a glossary of terms and more time getting folks into homes, or houses, or permanent living situations, or whatever you want to call them.

And it gets even more ridiculous when we get into the topic of gender. Here let me quote directly from columnist Nicholas Kristof.

> In an effort to be inclusive, the American Cancer Society recommends cancer screenings for "individuals with a cervix," the Centers for Disease Control and Prevention offers guidance "for breastfeeding people" and Cleveland Clinic offers advice for "people who menstruate."
>
> The aim is to avoid dehumanizing anyone. But some women feel dehumanized when referred to as "birthing

people," or when *The Lancet* had a cover about "bodies with vaginas."[10]

I guarantee you, when I met my wife, if I had gone up to her and told her she was one beautiful "birthing person," she would not be my wife today.

Or when I was doing my training, if somebody told me that we couldn't call fieldwork fieldwork anymore (because it could be associated with slavery or migrant labor), and instead I was participating in a *practicum*, I would have had no idea what you were talking about. How can we understand each other if we're prohibited from using words we all know?

Even if you want to support minorities, you can't call them that. The American Medical Association says that better terms would be "oppressed and "historically minoritized."[11]

For goodness' sake, if the goal is to unite or educate, this is not the way to do it. To solve a problem, you have to call it out. When you start using language nobody understands, you make it a lot harder to actually go after the root issue.

Now look, language changes over the years. There are words we don't use now that people used to use all the time. There's a natural evolution. But as the journalist George Packer points out, there's nothing organic about this change.[12] This is a revolution being foisted upon America by a small group of activist elites. They run organizations with names like the Center for Assessment and Policy Development and World Trust Educational Services. I've gone and looked at these organizations so that you don't have to. I can describe these organizations in lots of

> **To solve a problem, you have to call it out. When you start using language nobody understands, you make it a lot harder to actually go after the root issue.**

ways: well-intentioned, activist, misguided (in my view). They are not reflective of where the majority—or even, frankly, a minority (there's that word again, I hope I'm using it correctly)—of Americans are. And yet, this very small number of people is responsible for a large number of the "rules" that we now must follow when we talk or write.

One of my goals with this book is to better help us understand each other, to better help us communicate with each other. These language guides do the opposite. They create barriers. They create tests.

For example, the San Francisco Board of Supervisors replaced the word *felon* with "justice involved person."[13] Can we get real for a moment here? If you're a felon, you're a felon. If you're a rapist, you're not a justice-involved person, you're a rapist. If you're a murderer, you're not a justice-involved person, you're a murderer. If you're a tax cheat, you're not a justice-involved person, you're a tax cheat. You are what you are, so what's the use in all of us using some mealymouthed new phrase to deny it? How do we talk to the rape *victim* now? Do we tell her she wasn't raped? Do we tell her she just had an encounter with a justice-involved person? Who is being helped by this absurdity? I promise you, if someone is applying for a job and the application indicates they have been "justice involved" and the interviewer does not bother to track those details down, a village somewhere is missing their idiot! (I'm sure that expression is somehow an affront to either villages or idiots.)

Again, George Packer argues (and I agree with him) that words like that are more than a language change; it's actually an ideological claim. If someone is a justice-involved person, it says we're not going to use the specific word for what you did, because we think there's something illegitimate about the judicial system: the laws, the courts, the prisons. I've spent a lot of time helping clients navigate the judicial system, and that system may be a lot of things—slow, intimidating, confusing. But one thing it is *not* is illegitimate.

So, none of this solves a problem. But there is something the language police do achieve. They succeed in creating a test—a language test. A secret password to the "woke speakeasy." They give people a way to signal their virtue without having to engage in any of the behaviors we would call virtuous.

And do you know who would be the first person to fail this test? Thurgood Marshall, the first Black Supreme Court justice. The man who successfully argued before the Supreme Court that there's no such thing as "separate but equal." Why would this decorated civil rights leader fail the test? Because he spent a lot of time saying that he didn't want to be called "black." He wanted to use the term *Negro*, with a capital *N*. As a general rule, if Thurgood Marshall was wrong, we have to ask what exactly it takes to be right. In fact, back in the 1980s, when Rev. Jesse Jackson started encouraging people to use the term *African American*, Marshall decided not to. In his words, "It's everyone on his own. It's like what the old lady said when she kissed the cow—everyone to his own liking." I've heard a lot of country stories, but I don't know the one about the old lady and the cow. What I do know is that Marshall, in his wisdom, got at a very important point: we've traded rigid tests for basic reason, and that leads nowhere good fast.[14]

Everything I have written about in the last several pages I consider to be dangerous manipulations regarding free speech—using catastrophic language to describe things that aren't catastrophes, changing words, policing language, avoiding "triggers." But there's one manipulation that may be more dangerous than all of them, which is the redefinition of what constitutes hate speech.

We know that in this country, free speech is protected, by and large.

Even hateful speech, by and large, is protected.

However, hate speech that threatens serious bodily harm or causes an imminent breach of the peace is *not* protected.[15]

But activists and agitators succeeded in redefining a subset of speech as "hate speech." And not just your run-of-the-mill hate speech, which is already hard to argue should be protected. After all, it is unkind, ungenerous, uncivilized, ugly.

But now we're talking about speech that is "assaultive conduct."

Now it can be regulated, shut down, prosecuted.

And, again, there's no problem with that—speech that incites people to lawlessness, or presents a true threat, should be shut down.

The problem is how broadly the activists want to define it.

If you express a desire to have a say in deciding who comes across our border, you're guilty of "hate speech."

If you want to say that sex differences are written in the chromosomes and can't be changed with hormone therapy or sex reassignment surgery, you're guilty of "hate speech."

If you want to say that the most qualified person should get the job or be admitted to the college independent of race, you're guilty of "hate speech."

And while it may not get you arrested, it can sure get you muzzled or fired.

Because statements like that are now deemed "assaultive conduct" that cause harm.

That's why we're seeing so many college professors disciplined, suspended, or fired. Activists said the language they used, the words they chose, were hurtful, assaultive.

In the near future, it *could* get you arrested, at least in Michigan. As I write this, a bill was passed by the Michigan House of Representatives that would make it a felony to intimidate someone with words.[16] The bill, which may or may not become law, would allow for Michiganders to be fined ten thousand dollars and put in jail for up to five years if they cause someone to feel "terrorized, frightened, or threatened" by words, which could include using the wrong gender pronouns.

When I look at all of these things that are now considered assault, all I can think is that the real assault, of course, is on reason.

POLL RESPONSE

In the last year, have you struggled to remember the "right" word you're supposed to use to describe someone or something in a way you consider to be sensitive, in a situation or a conversation that might be sensitive?

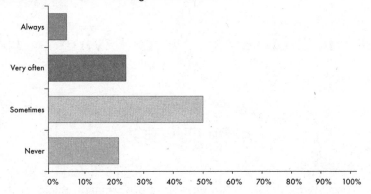

My point in posing this question is, we should all struggle to be sensitive to other people and their feelings. What we shouldn't be is afraid that we're going to be attacked or labeled a hater or phobic because of a slip of the tongue. We all make honest mistakes. I encourage people to look at the individual's pattern of behavior, not what they might say in a given moment. Maybe they had a lapse, or maybe they hadn't caught up with that new evolution of language. Which is why I say we need a counsel culture, not a cancel culture. Let's find out what's really in people's hearts. Maybe they just need some enlightenment, maybe they need some conversation about it. What they don't need is to be humiliated in the town square because of a slip of the tongue, or because they used a word that they weren't aware could be offensive to someone's sensibilities.

CHAPTER 4

It's the 2020s, but We're Living in *1984*

POLL QUESTION

How often do you feel that you are being told the truth by an "assigned authority"—an unelected government official such as the head of an agency?

- ☐ Always
- ☐ Very often
- ☐ Sometimes
- ☐ Never

I must have been in the seventh or eighth grade when I first read George Orwell's haunting novel *1984*. I have since read it several times and it gets more and more relevant, more and more disturbing, each time.

When I first read it at the age of twelve or thirteen, I thought it was just really well-written science fiction. I wasn't mature enough to appreciate that it was based on the realities of Stalin's Soviet Union and the horrors of Nazi Germany.

But I did understand that it was a commentary on how a totalitarian dictatorship can manipulate the collective consciousness of an entire society if it can completely control the flow and content of the information people receive.

I promised you a book, not a book report, but bear with me for a minute, because the parallels are creepy, and the warning is relevant.

In Orwell's world, the superstate "Oceania" is led by "Big Brother" and his political party, a cultish band of adherents. The populace has to deal with the Party's "Thought Police" and "Ministry of Truth." Surveillance is ubiquitous. People are denied any freedom of thought or speech. If they run afoul of the rules, they can be erased, vaporized, disappeared, turned into an "unperson."

In the book, we see people become so programmed that they *want* to be told what words to use and what to think. They want choices made for them, because it takes away any pressure to think for themselves, or fear of what might happen if you do.

For example, listen to one of the characters who is assigned to police language, and to get people to use what is called "Newspeak." "We're destroying words—scores of them, hundreds of them, every day . . . do you know that Newspeak is the only language in the world whose vocabulary gets smaller every year."

Sound familiar?

Or consider another concept from Orwell's terrifyingly prescient book, "doublethink." Doublethink is described as the ability "to hold simultaneously two opinions which cancelled out, knowing them to be contradictory and believing in both of them."

Think about all the times we see someone today doing the opposite of what they claim to be doing. Let me give you an example: President Joe Biden's Inflation Reduction Act. This was a law that will do a lot of things. But one thing most serious analysts agree on is that it will not meaningfully reduce inflation.[1]

And just so you know that I'm not putting my thumb on the political scale, it's not just Democrats. Consider George W. Bush's Healthy Forests Restoration Act. How did that law create "healthy forests"? By allowing more timber harvesting on federally protected land.

Or consider, as I noted earlier, that as I write this, Democrats *and* Republicans in Congress came together to raise our nation's debt ceiling above $31.4 trillion—allowing us to owe *more* than $31 trillion—with a bill that they named, wait for it, the Fiscal Responsibility Act.[2]

And it's not just governmental authority. Look at how we have reframed an obesity epidemic (that affects nearly 20 percent of children in America)[3] and that we know will have significant lifelong health consequences—heart disease, breathing problems, joint problems, gallstones, anxiety and depression, greater risk of stroke, many types of cancer—some pretty negative outcomes.[4] So how are we going to handle it? By embracing "body positivity." It really is Orwellian when you think about it.

Another parallel? In May 2022 the Biden administration actually implemented something called the Disinformation Governance Board (DGB) as part of the Department of Homeland Security. I was so glad to see that many people from both sides of the political aisle were so outraged that they had to decommission the DGB before it ever really got started. Almost everyone drew a direct parallel to Orwell's *1984* Ministry of Truth.

> And then, of course, there's Orwell's famous term—*unperson.* Someone who disappears because they ran afoul of Big Brother's rules in some way. Today we'd simply call it "cancelled."

And then, of course, there's Orwell's famous term—*unperson.* Someone who disappears because they ran afoul of Big Brother's rules in some way. Today we'd simply call it "cancelled."

Being cancelled is when you say or do the wrong thing, or post the wrong thing on social media, and the mob comes for you. All of a sudden you're fired from your job, excluded from your friend group, alienated from family members, your kids get mocked in school. It's like you've been put on the sex offender registry, and your picture is nailed to every telephone pole in the neighborhood. Nobody wants to be an unperson, so sometimes you stay in a scary group or a scary belief system, because the only thing scarier is being kicked out of the group or having to develop your own beliefs.

I may have less hair than I did, and my tie might not be as wide, but it sure feels like *1984* to me. Perhaps America's greatest and most valid claim to fame is that we are the "Land of the Free." Why then would we elicit, maintain, or even allow such a cancer to infect our society?

Why would we bend to anyone (or any group) whose only tactic is relentless, insidious indoctrination punctuated by guilt induction and threats of public humiliation for noncompliance and independent thought?

All with the goal of gradually altering the beliefs and values of individuals or groups.

As we'll discuss in greater depth, the internet in general and social platforms in particular have been a force multiplier in the ability to both seduce and intimidate. These fringe groups using mental manipulation of individuals and other groups instill a distorted worldview, eroding reason and causing people to blindly adopt harmful and false theories. It may sound dramatic, but I see these fringe groups wrapping their tentacles around the minds of the unwary, warping their perceptions, and replacing truth with a manipulative, self-serving fiction.

Deceitful language becomes weaponized to propagate unfounded, scientifically contradicted ideas and theories until they take root in the public consciousness, like a spider expertly weaving a web of lies, trapping its prey in a maze of confusion and cognitive dissonance that keeps them from ever questioning the baseless dogmas they are now being fed. We must be discerning. Even a dumb cow knows to swallow grass and spit out weeds. Shouldn't we hold ourselves to at least that standard?

POLL RESPONSE

How often do you feel that you are being told the truth by an"assigned authority"—an unelected government official such as the head of an agency?

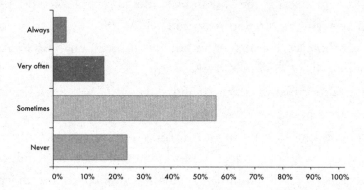

I was interested in asking this question because I'm concerned that unelected officials, in particular, have overstepped their authority in several areas, one of which we'll talk about when we discuss our nation's COVID response. It seems a lot of you agree it's unelected officials that are wielding so much power. Not the people you cast your vote for, but people that are running agencies and dictating a lot of policy in our daily living. We didn't elect these people, but they sure have a lot of power in our lives. How much do we believe them, how much power do they hold, and how much do we question them?

CHAPTER 5

The Dangers of Rewriting

POLL QUESTION

Is there a book you loved as a child that you can't find any-more because it's been withdrawn from the market, or a book that's been removed from your child's school library because it's "no longer appropriate"?

☐ Yes

☐ No

Crack open one of the books you loved reading to your child these days and you may find that there have been some . . . well, changes.

Books, especially children's books, are being revised and rewritten left and right to satisfy the demands of—who exactly? I'll tell you, at least what I was able to figure out.

I defy you to find me a single person who, upon reading *The Adventures of Huckleberry Finn*, decided that they were going to start using the word *Injun* in daily conversation.

I defy you to find me someone who thought it was okay to use the N-word because a character in a book that was published in the 1880s did. In fact, I would argue that seeing those words in those outdated circumstances is what teaches us that we don't talk like that today.

Well, thank goodness we've ended that epidemic, because you won't find those words in the book anymore. In fact, someone reading the book today would never even know they were there. Nobody will run the risk of being hurt by a word that someone used 140 years ago. That's a good thing, right?

I don't think so.

By editing the book, the woke mob entirely *misses the point* of the book. And I don't know about you, but I don't need them protecting me. *The Adventures of Huckleberry Finn* is supposed to be a satire of the racism of the time. What made it revolutionary was the fact that it was written not with fancy-pants language and seventy-five-cent words—it was written in the language people spoke, with regional words and variations. When it was released, it was criticized for using the very words that are now being erased!

That's the problem. Books become classics because of the writer or artist's vision. And now, in the name of protecting feelings, we have people messing with that vision. Again, no thank you, I don't need you protecting me. I can think for myself. I don't need you protecting my children. They can think for themselves, and as a parent, I can help them do that. We don't need you as moral gatekeepers. We don't need you, and even if we did, you have demonstrated you are not qualified.

Consider another childhood favorite, Dr. Seuss's first book, *And to Think That I Saw It on Mulberry Street*. It's about a boy who, on his way home from school, imagines increasingly ridiculous things he wants to tell his father he saw. Unfortunately, he imagines seeing "a Chinese man" with chopsticks, a "Rajah, with rubies," and two characters who seem to be Inuit (which is the word we now use for Eskimo) being pulled by reindeer. Well, that's tough sledding for all of us—because these depictions, we are now told, are "hurtful and wrong."

So, the world loses a sweet book about the power of imagination because we can't differentiate caricature from reality?

Those who defend the changes say, look, even Dr. Seuss updated some of his stuff to keep up with the times, so why shouldn't we?

Actually, there are a couple of reasons.

First, because he was the artist—he's allowed to mess with his own art.

Second, because I'm more scared of the slippery slope than the words and images in those books.

> **Book editing is the first step on the way to wholesale book altering, which might even be more dangerous than book banning.**

Book editing is the first step on the way to wholesale book altering, which might even be more dangerous than book banning.

Would it be appropriate to write a book today the way some of those books were written decades ago? That's the choice of the author and the publisher. It certainly wouldn't be consistent with the mores and folkways of our time, so probably not. But to bend the reality of what happened generations ago is deceptive to young people today and robs them of the chance to understand how we have evolved as a society. (And it often robs kids of the very things they enjoyed about the book to begin with.)

When someone says that we've made no progress, that we're right where we were in the 1940s and '50s and '60s, the answer is no, we're not. And for proof, we look at books and movies and say, "We don't use words like that today, we don't say things like that today, we don't have the same attitudes today."

So, do some of these changes, on some level, make sense? Sure, you can argue over this word or that word. But you start changing history and rewriting literature, you are walking in dress shoes on a dangerously slippery slope. How long until you write out entire characters? Or change the plot to conform to whatever the mob wants today?

How long until someone says, "Look, the world hasn't changed one bit since the 1950s," because the book they *think* is from that time was actually updated just this year? My position is if we change history, we are lying to an entire generation about what took place before they were born.

Stuff happened or it didn't.

We used different words.

Learn it. Understand it. A story can be a great story and help you recognize the ways in which we've grown and changed.

Because once you open the door to one change, you open the door to a million others. And if you think I'm being ridiculous about the slippery slope that we risk getting on, I regret to inform you that we're already on it.

Maybe you remember reading Roald Dahl's classics—either yourself or to your children.

Charlie and the Chocolate Factory, *The Big Friendly Giant*, *James and the Giant Peach*. Classics. But also, pretty dark and creepy. In fact, that's why a lot of kids love them.

Do you remember Augustus Gloop from *Charlie and the Chocolate Factory*? If you do, what's the one word you would use to describe him? Probably *fat*.

Not anymore, because that word is no longer used. We can't call a character whose central characteristic is his greed and gluttony a common word that is often the result of greed and gluttony?

Oompa Loompas, who were once described as "small men," have now become "small people." Thank God we've finally struck a blow for gender equality among a fictitious race of people.

The list goes on, and on, and on.

One retroactive change that hit close to home for me was in Dahl's

The Witches. The witches move through their world in costume. It is later revealed in a dramatic scene that when they take off their wigs, they are all bald.

But now if you read the book, at the terrifying moment that the witches reveal who they truly are, there's a new line in the book that says: "There are plenty of other reasons why women might wear wigs and there is certainly nothing wrong with that."

No kidding. This is a story, not a public service announcement.

I guarantee every little girl reading that book has tried on a costume with a wig.

Nobody in the book is saying that wigs are wrong or that a woman in a wig is evil or that a wig always hides something sinister. Only by adding that stupid extra line would a child even think to think that.

As someone who might be described as "hair-challenged," I can't understand why that line needs to be changed. The author is telling you that not all is always what it appears to be. Guess what, that's a pretty good life lesson!

One of the authors who has become frustrated watching his publisher change his writing right under his nose is RL Stine, the author of the wildly successful *Goosebumps* series. Throughout his books, weight references such as having "at least six chins," resembling "a bowling ball," and having "squirrel cheeks" have been stripped away.

It looks like in children's books these days, there's one form of representation that isn't allowed. Apparently, nobody is allowed to be fat. That seems to be a pretty strange line to draw at a time when nearly 20 percent of children in America are categorized as obese.[1]

Obesity is a public health crisis. It's often a mental health crisis as well. And children being cruel to other children because of it is *reality*. Yes, we need to deal with the health crisis. Yes, we need to deal with bullying and name-calling. But making sure that childhood obesity and all of the issues surrounding it gets erased or woke-washed accomplishes absolutely nothing other than altering an author's original vision.

We see something similar in Stine's book *Don't Go to Sleep!* Stine's editors changed a scene where a boy dismisses Tolstoy's *Anna Karenina* as "girl's stuff." The boy now insists it's simply "not interesting." Look, books appeal to kids because they meet them in their reality. And the reality is that for as long as there have been boys, they'll sometimes say that something is "girl's stuff." They're saying some things appeal more to one gender than the other. And you know what? They do.

With this edit, the nameless publishers have made sure that *every child* gets the message that Tolstoy is boring. That doesn't seem like a win to me.

In a lot of these cases, the edits are coming from a group called Inclusive Minds. Inclusive Minds is an organization that takes great pains to say that they do not rewrite or edit texts; they simply "help identify language and portrayals that could be inauthentic or problematic, and to highlight why, as well as indicate potential solutions." These suggestions come from their "inclusion ambassadors"—who "can share nuances related to their lived experience."

That may be true. They may not rewrite or edit texts.

But it is also true that they "encourage" book creators to hire them to consult on the books they're releasing or rereleasing. And it's also true that Inclusive Minds has "campaigned" against books that are not inclusive.

All of a sudden, it starts to feel a little like a shakedown, doesn't it? Hire us and we'll make sure your book gets our seal of approval. And once it gets our seal of approval, you have a get-out-of-jail-free card for when the mob comes after you.

Who are the people behind Inclusive Minds? I have no idea. There's not a single individual's name on their entire website. That's a warning sign.

And a lot of publishers are willing to buy that card. And a lot of people want to flash that card.

It's almost like they're selling woke insurance. But what they're really doing is just providing woke-washing! All we really need is just some commonsense perspective.

Do some of these books use words we don't use anymore? Yup.

Do they sometimes espouse values we don't hold anymore? Also yup.

But our job is to read them and—in reading them—understand why we don't use those words or espouse those values anymore.

Because we are throwing the baby out with the bathwater, at best.

And at worst, we're putting ourselves in a place where every book is being published in *1984*, when truth is decided by whoever is in charge.

And that, to use a word that the good folks at Inclusive Minds would surely demand I change—because they've demanded that other authors change it—is crazy. I don't think you need a group of outside consultants to change this book, because I think you understand that *crazy* is a term that has plenty of other valid definitions, such as excitement, infatuated, or "crazy good," and that I would never use it in a clinical setting to describe a patient or their behavior or thinking.

POLL RESPONSE

Is there a book you loved as a child, that you can't find anymore because it's been withdrawn from the market, or a book that's been removed from your child's school library because it's no "longer appropriate"?

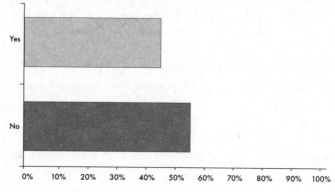

By the way, when I looked at the people with children still at home who responded to this question, the number of people answering "yes" jumped up quite a bit. This concerns me.

PART TWO

From What They're Doing to What You're Doing

I've spent the last several chapters showing how and what a small group of fringe thinkers are doing to us—making us fear saying the wrong thing, making us change the words we use and the words we read, convincing us that words as much as weapons can cause harm.

In the next section, we're going to turn from what others are doing to us to what we're doing to ourselves.

But before we do that, I want to answer the question you've probably had in your head since the beginning: Why?

Why are they doing this? And why are we allowing it?

Let's start with why they are doing it.

Some answers can be found in the work of Jonathan Haidt, a social psychologist at New York University, and Greg Lukianoff, the president and CEO of the Foundation for Individual Rights and Expression (FIRE). Their book *The Coddling of the American Mind* is in my opinion one of the most important books to come out in recent years.*

They write about two trends that are colliding right now and supercharging cancel culture and the Tyranny of the Fringe.

The first is that, as they write, "social media makes it extraordinarily easy to join crusades, express solidarity and outrage, and to shun traitors."[1] Basically, it makes it very easy to toss gasoline on a fire. And it makes it easy for that "fire" to be seen by lots of people, people who are looking for that "exciting new club" to make them feel connected, relevant, involved in the "happening thing."

All it takes is a click to "Like, Follow, or Subscribe!" and you are

---

* It has practically become a bible among HR professionals, who are struggling to figure out the challenges of working with a new generation.

"IN"! You are part of something bigger than yourself. You might wake up in the morning feeling left out, directionless, and without a purpose or reference group. By the end of the day, after a few clicks and shares and reading and internalizing some dubious claims, you are part of an action group!

When you think about it, that alone explains a lot. In the past, if you wanted to join a cause, you'd have to show up at a meeting, paint signs, get people to sign a paper petition, and deliver it somewhere. And doing all that made you slow down and think about whether you were *really* outraged enough to jump into action that way. Now all you need to do is tap a screen or click a mouse.

> **And, what's worse, as I've said before, is that offense has become "medicalized," meaning that someone is now considered actually hurt or injured by what was said. It's no longer an opinion. It's an assault.**

The second trend is that the idea of offensiveness has changed. As Haidt and Lukianoff write, "A claim that someone's words are 'offensive' is not just an expression of one's own subjective feeling of 'offendedness.' It is, rather, a public charge that the speaker has done something objectively wrong."

And, what's worse, as I've said before, is that offense has become "medicalized," meaning that someone is now considered actually hurt or injured by what was said. It's no longer an opinion. It's an assault.

And because it's an assault, schools and workplaces need to take it seriously. All of a sudden, people need to say, "This is the intentional infliction of emotional distress. This could result in suicide, we have to deal with this." So, what happens? A bunch of professors and coaches and bosses get called onto the carpet and get suspended or fired because their words triggered feelings of inadequacy or feelings of trauma, or feelings of lack of safety. Instead of the rewards of learning how to be resilient, people are instead *rewarded* for entitled behavior.

To make matters worse, a lot of the people claiming offense aren't hurt at all—physically or emotionally. They're getting offended on someone else's behalf. And as I wrote about earlier, oftentimes they don't even care about whether you're really antagonistic to the cause; what they care about is that they caught someone misspeaking. The new version of being caught red-handed is being caught with the wrong word in your mouth. Intent doesn't matter. What matters is that you can be hauled into the town square and publicly flogged because it serves an activist agenda.

The people who throw these labels around tend not to care what you actually think and feel. Instead, they want to engage in what the journalist Jonathan Rauch called the "offendedness sweepstakes."[2] If you can claim offense and, better yet, claim that you've been offended by a high-profile company, or celebrity, or politician, or athlete, or historical figure, you can ride the coattails of that controversy to get a lot of attention and free media coverage, to fundraising success, maybe even to celebrity yourself.

Put simply, joining the mob is easier than ever, and leading the mob is more rewarding than ever. What's not to like? Now that we know why they're doing it, the next question is, why do we allow it?

Why would any single one of us, anyone with a speck of healthy skepticism or an appreciation for the value of scientific validation and verification, allow this Tyranny of the Fringe to get so much as a toehold, let alone drive a narrative that totally ignores the psychosocial principles we know work in maintaining cohesion, motivation, proper development, and mental and physical health? Why would we allow anyone to advance theories and practices ignoring verified truths in history, biology, or science in general?

Before you read another word, take a moment to pause and

answer that question in writing. Don't just ponder it and move on. Really think about it. What is holding you back, shutting you down, and shutting you up? What do you see that you aren't saying? What are you afraid of?

In this section, we're going to talk about all those things you wrote down, and what we can do about them.

CHAPTER 6

Deprogram Yourself,
Because the Truth Is Out There

POLL QUESTION

Think of any interest group that you either support or oppose—pro- or anti-gun, pro- or anti-abortion, pro– or anti–transgender rights, Black Lives Matter, or Blue Lives Matter. How often do you think the spokespeople for those interest groups reflect the beliefs, feelings, and attitudes of the overall group?

☐ Always

☐ Very often

☐ Sometimes

☐ Never

Now, you may notice that I'm using the word *deprogram* here, a word that most often applies to cults. I do that purposefully.

I'm not saying that you're going to sign up to follow the next Jim Jones, the cult leader who convinced more than nine hundred of his followers to commit mass suicide at his campground in Guyana. You're not going to fall under the spell of the next Charles Manson, who ordered his Manson family followers to commit murder. In fact, you're more likely to be wondering how anyone could ever join a cult to begin with.

That's never the intention, but what if I told you that you might already be involved in something questionable, something designed to suck you in, take your time, take your money, and erase your individuality? Everywhere we turn, people, companies, political parties, and media platforms are using cultlike tactics to ensure you become a believer. And I want to make sure that you're being who you are on purpose, which means understanding—and resisting—the ways in which you might be programmed.

One of my good friends is Rick Alan Ross, who leads the non-profit Cult Education Institute. He points out that the one core characteristic of a destructive cult is "an absolute authoritarian leader who is always right, who is the defining element and driving force of the group and who becomes an object of worship."

It's important to recognize that nobody is always right.

No person is deserving of your total worship.

But in cultlike environments, you're not getting any accurate feedback.

This is something that has been with us through time. Think about the Hans Christian Andersen folktale "The Emperor's New Clothes." The way the original story goes, two swindlers promise to weave the emperor a beautiful set of new clothes. But the catch is that the clothes will be invisible to people who are stupid. When officials go visit the weavers at work and see nothing, they pretend to see something. "What fine clothes!" they say, not wanting to be exposed as fools. Finally, when the emperor parades through town in his new clothes, which was really just his birthday suit, it's a child—an innocent—who points out that the emperor is wearing nothing at all. The desire to go along, to not stir the pot, to be accepted is incredibly powerful.

Call it a cult. Call it gaslighting. Call it the Fox News, CNN, or MSNBC effect. But there are some warning signs that you can spot that will allow you to deprogram yourself, the same way cult deprogrammers help remove people from cults. One thing I want you to recognize is that when you try to remove someone from a cult, they often get defensive. You're telling them that they've given up their power and made a poor decision. You don't have to be defensive, because this is a conversation you're having only with yourself, not someone else who is accusing you of being brainwashed. I'm going to pose some questions to you now. Answer these as honestly as you possibly can. To do that, take a moment and resolve to take a really hard look at how you may have become overly affiliated with any group you now consider yourself a member of. I say that not knowing whether you are a Democrat, Republican, or an independent. The same standards hold true for everyone. But remember, winners deal with the truth. They have the courage to be straight with themselves even if it's painful.

> ➤ Did you feel "love-bombed" at the beginning—were you told how smart and wise you were? The group leaders or recruiters really made you feel wanted.

> ➤ Do you like them primarily because they like you?

> ➤ Is this group that you're part of open to criticism? Can they ever admit being wrong? Do you ever hear them say anything like "We have to admit, the other side has a really good point there"?

> ➤ Does an issue agenda start to feel like a religion? Does it feel like you'd almost be "excommunicated" if you asked questions or expressed doubt?

> ➤ Did you come to a conclusion on one issue, but now find yourself being asked to believe in related things that have you feeling less comfortable?

➤ Do you find that you're cutting off or being cut off from other sources of input, information, or commentary?

➤ Do you find yourself growing more distant from people to whom you'd been close for a long time, like friends and family?

➤ Does it feel emotionally painful to dial back or step away, almost like loneliness or grief?

If you answered yes to any of these questions, you've given more of yourself than you should to others, and you need to make sure you're operating in the realm of reason, the realm of truth.

Because that's the first and most basic way in which you might be "programmed"—by a simple inability to distinguish truth from fiction.

The Truth Is Out There

What is the most basic question you can ask when presented with a piece of information? "Is this true?"

We've all heard the saying from Mark Twain that a lie can travel around the world and back while the truth is still lacing up its boots.* Today we know exactly how true that is. A couple of professors at the Massachusetts Institute of Technology did a study where they looked at over 100,000 news stories that had been tweeted by 3 million people over 4 million times—and they found that lies traveled six times faster than the truth.[1]

---

* Ironically, even that saying is sort of a lie, because the real saying comes from a writer in the 1700s, Jonathan Swift, who said, "Falsehood flies, and the truth comes limping after it." https://www.politifact.com/factchecks/2017/oct/09/colin-kaepernick/nfls-colin -kaepernick-incorrectly-credits-winston-/.

I want you to read how they summarized their study, because I can't say it better myself:

> Falsehood diffused significantly farther, faster, deeper, and more broadly than the truth in all categories of information, and the effects were more pronounced for false political news than for false news about terrorism, natural disasters, science, urban legends, or financial information. We found that false news was more novel than true news, which suggests that people were more likely to share novel information. . . . Contrary to conventional wisdom, robots accelerated the spread of true and false news at the same rate, implying that false news spreads more than the truth because humans, not robots, are more likely to spread it.[2]

Listen to what they're telling us here—one of the reasons that lies travel faster is because they sound "newer" and more interesting. And you know this. The truth is messy. There aren't always clearly defined heroes and villains. If a story seems too neat and tidy to be true, it probably is.

And if I choose to believe the lie, or spread it, I'm not thinking or behaving rationally.

When you hear something or are about to share something, take a breath and think: "Is this thought I'm having, is this emotional, is it hearsay, is it just something that's being touted in the media, or have I verified this?"

Is it factual, empirical, verifiable information?

The truth is messy. There aren't always clearly defined heroes and villains. If a story seems too neat and tidy to be true, it probably is.

If it's not, stop immediately.

That's a discontinuation criterion: I've got false information here. I need to wait until I can get verifiable information I know is accurate. Real journalists used to do that. Now, unfortunately, a premium is too often placed on being first rather than factual.

This book is intended to be a blueprint for how you can be all that I believe American society needs you to be in order to flourish in this time when we have an awful lot of people, factions, and entities standing up and yelling, "Hey! Over here! Forget what you thought you knew, what you held dear and relied on, and come follow us. Come on! Forget that you believe it is light during the day and dark at night. We have new answers, real answers, and *we* love you. We love and accept and include everybody!"

That's the "love bomb" messaging; that's the beginning of the "gaslighting." You of course can easily test the authenticity of it all in two easy steps:

1. Dare to question the premise of what they are promoting. Just say something like "Wow! You know what, that does not seem right to me but hey, I'm open-minded. Just tell me how do you account for decades of verified scientific findings that contradict what you are saying about (fill in the blank)."

2. Flatly reject what is being promoted by saying something like "I'm sorry but I *know* what you are advocating is patently false and in fact dangerous so I cannot support that agenda." Then add, "I hope we can just agree to disagree and still be friends and our children can still play together."

Odds are pretty good you are going to find out that "we love and accept everyone" message will quickly be replaced with "You are a hater, a bigot, a racist"—whatever character assassination label fits the subject matter of the moment. Why? People pushing ideas or positions that lack a solid underpinning or factual basis tend to get very defensive very fast when challenged. Why? Because they have no answers. Their only choice is to "change the game" and stop talking about the subject and start talking about you.

It is an effective strategy, because no one likes to be criticized, held up to public ridicule, or judged harshly—regardless of who is doing the judging. It is almost always easier to "go along to get along," because then at least people aren't hurling insults, tweeting ugly sentiments about you, writing your place of employment to make sure they know what a horrible person they have on staff, or excluding you from block parties or backyard barbecues.

Avoiding getting caught in the current is not easy, and those attempting to control you know it, whether the issue is who you vote for, school curriculums, crime and punishment, positions on how to respond to an influx of homeless, transgender issues, abortion, strategies to control school shootings, safe zones for drug addicts, climate change—whatever the subject of the moment is.

So, you have a decision to make. Are you going to take the easy, compliant route or are you going to take the more honest, authentic, but sometimes more difficult route?

That more difficult route is the one where you decide to be who you are and live your life that way: consciously, mindfully, on purpose. That means you may need a blueprint to deprogram yourself. To stop answering questions the way someone else wants you to answer them. To stop buying into a worldview that you don't embrace, or playing into a conversation that you don't want to have. It's easier said than done, I know.

That's why I want you to ask yourself a very basic question: Who do I want to be, and where do I want to go?

POLL RESPONSE

Think of any interest group that you either support or oppose—pro- or anti-gun, pro- or anti-abortion, pro– or anti–transgender rights, Black Lives Matter, or Blue Lives Matter. How often do you think the spokespeople for those interest groups reflect the beliefs, feelings, and attitudes of the overall group?

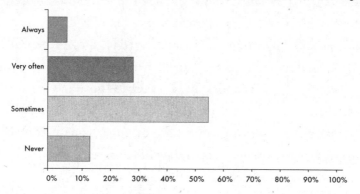

Part of why I wanted to see your response to this question is that I've always felt that at a certain point, group leaders begin running their own personal agendas. The most valuable currency to them is attention, and so they stake out increasingly extreme positions in order to get it.

The majority of individuals polled answered "Sometimes" or "Often." Now, that's enough to make us wonder, at least ask, are these spokespeople running their own agenda, or do they really represent the group they supposedly represent? And I would caution all of us that the more radical and more extreme the spokesperson seems to be, the more we should question whether the entire group is that radical and extreme.

CHAPTER 7

We're Doing Our Enemies' Work for Them

POLL QUESTION

Once you have formed an opinion about something of importance, how likely are you to revisit that opinion and seek out or seriously consider new information?

- ☐ Always
- ☐ Very often
- ☐ Sometimes
- ☐ Never

Recently, the most important document you've never heard of landed in my inbox.

It was sent to me by my good friend and colleague Chase Hughes, a twenty-year Navy veteran. Later in this book, I write about the importance of developing what I call "consequential knowledge," a skill set that you work to acquire that is of special value. The skill set that the world can't do without. The skill set that can't be replicated by grabbing someone off the street and training them for a few hours. Boy oh boy, is Chase Hughes the perfect example of that guiding

principle! During his time in the Navy, he became focused on better ways of conducting intelligence operations—we're talking about
everything from recruiting foreign assets to sophisticated and effica-
cious techniques for interrogating enemy combatants. He created
behavior-profiling tools and manuals to "read" humans and influence
their behavior. It's an impressive, hard-earned, and harder-to-replicate
set of skills and knowledge. You ain't going to find it in your average
bear or even your not-so-average one.

After his service in the military, he took everything he learned
to the private sector and began advising government agencies, police
groups, and other organizations on behavior science. He also wrote
bestselling books on persuasion, influence, and behavior profiling.

Chase had received the document he sent me in the original Russian, and he then had it translated. It was a "tradecraft manual on
psychopolitics."

Psychopolitics, it says on the first page, is "the art and science of
asserting and maintaining dominion over the thoughts and loyalties
of individuals, officers, bureaus, and masses, and the effecting of the
conquest of enemy nations through 'mental healing.'"

In short, it's a guide to brainwashing a nation. It's a long-term
plan to brainwash, demoralize, and thereby destroy an entire nation.
We have to remember that a lot of early work in psychology, such as
the research on classical conditioning, was done by Ivan Pavlov, a Russian and Soviet psychologist, in the late 1800s. The Russians are not
new to the arena.

And I hate to tell you, what they're talking about in this manual
on psychopolitics, well, let's just say it's effective.

How do I know this? Because it's working, on us, right now.[1]

As Chase told me when I asked him about it, "I'm literally a brainwashing expert, and they [the Russians] are doing it."[2]

In 1984 (there's that year again!), a former KGB agent named
Yuri Alexandrovich Bezmenov, who had defected to Canada, gave an

interview in which he described a process that is outlined *exactly* in the document that Chase sent me. It's a terrifying interview, and you can watch it yourself.*

The goal, according to both the guide and Bezmenov, is ideological subversion, "to change the perception of reality of every American to such an extent that despite the abundance of information no one is able to come to sensible conclusions in the interest of defending themselves, their families, their community, and their country."[3]

Step one in this effort is demoralization. A "demoralized" person is, according to Yuri, "programmed to think and react to certain stimuli in a certain pattern. You cannot change their mind even if you expose them to authentic information. Even if you prove that white is white and black is black, you still cannot change the basic perception and the logic of behavior . . . exposure to true information does not matter anymore. . . . A person who was demoralized is unable to assess true information. The facts tell nothing to him. Even if I shower him with information, with authentic proof, with documents, with pictures; even if I take him by force to the Soviet Union and show him [a] concentration camp, he will refuse to believe it. . . ."

According to Yuri, "the demoralization process in the United States is basically completed already." And he says it's been successful beyond what the KGB could dream. He adds, "And most of it is done *by* Americans *to* Americans. . . . Exposure to true information does not matter anymore."

Reading the guide and watching the interview are terrifying, because we're playing right into the hands of our enemies. We're demoralizing ourselves. And we need to break out of it. Here's how:

You've probably heard the old joke about the door-to-door salesman who's going through a neighborhood, and he sees a sign that says, "Democratic puppies for sale." A week later, he's back in the

---

* https://youtu.be/bX3EZCVj2XA.

same neighborhood, and the sign now says, "Republican puppies for sale." Curious, he knocks on the door, and when the homeowner opens it, he says, "How'd they go from being Democratic puppies to Republican puppies?" And the homeowner says, "Oh, their eyes are open now."

Look, it's not the best joke. And you can reverse it and make it a joke about Republicans. I don't really care. The point is that things can change when you open your eyes. As Chase and I discussed, one way to lessen a technique's power is to bring it into the light. The example he uses is when you're at an event and you're introduced to some alpha-male type. Instead of shaking your hand, he tries to assert his dominance by squeezing the life out of it, just a bone-crushing handshake. Chase's response: "Wow, that's a really powerful grip. A little bit painful, but I think you did a great job. You must be really powerful and strong." You can start to see why Chase is an expert at all kinds of countermeasures. Because that sounds like a compliment and feels like a compliment, but it totally neutralizes the power Mr. Alpha Male was trying to assert.

But even opening your eyes and pulling techniques into the light isn't enough. As Chase says, gaining awareness is not the same as gaining control. Awareness is necessary, but not sufficient. We need to gain control of our lives, our decisions, and our country.

As you're reading this, don't you wonder why this is not the focus of major headlines in newspapers and magazines across America? Think about all the things that are getting headlines and about the fact that America is under an ongoing subversive attack is getting none. This is reality and it is distressing. Putting me in a room with a box of puppies is not going make me feel any better about it.

Luckily, I don't want to gloss over it. I don't want to be made to feel better about it. I want to acknowledge it, talk about it, and deal with it. That is exactly why I am writing about it here.

POLL RESPONSE

Once you have formed an opinion about something of importance, how likely are you to revisit that opinion and seek out or seriously consider new information?

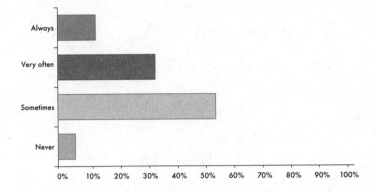

I would ask you to examine your answer to that and try to come up with a few examples where you have actually held a strong opinion, had it challenged, revisited it, and changed your position. I think we *think* we do more than we do. I think we need to challenge ourselves to reopen that data window and be sure we're not suffering from confirmation bias. That we're not looking only at data that reinforces what we think, feel, and believe. I don't want you to change an opinion that's based on fact, I'm just saying be open because I think we probably overevaluate our openness.

CHAPTER 8

Programmed by Algorithm
(You're Angry, They Profit)

POLL QUESTION

How often do you read a news report or see a tweet that makes you angry?

☐ Daily

☐ Weekly

☐ Monthly

☐ Never

If you're anything like me, you've heard of TikTok, and maybe you've seen some videos on the platform. But you don't really get it. That's okay, because I'm about to explain it to you, or, at the very least, demystify it. My team and I have done substantial digging and consulted with some world-class experts (special thanks to my good friend, cybersecurity expert, and creator of the wonderful site Bullyville.com, James McGibney), and my takeaway is this: you don't want to let Tik-Tok get within a country mile of your child's phone.

Let me explain why, in a way that assumes you know nothing

more about it than I did when I began the quest to figure things out, which was very little.

And by the way, even if you have never been on TikTok, I guarantee that every son, daughter, niece, nephew, and other young person in your life has—two-thirds of Americans between the ages of fourteen and twenty-four use it. It's an app where people can create and share all sorts of short videos: singing, dancing, comedy, lip-syncing, pranks, cooking—whatever. Generally, it seems pretty wholesome and innocent. I opened a TikTok account a few years ago to experience it from a user point of view and have found it very interesting. But there's definitely a dark underside to it.

And that's not just because TikTok is a Chinese company that can be used to spy on us and gather data on us, although there is that too.

The reason I say it is not the fun, wholesome, innocent entertainment site it appears to be is the content that gets served up and how and why that content gets presented to each specific user.

One of my newer friends and associates is Imran Ahmed, the founder and CEO of a nonprofit organization called the Center for Countering Digital Hate. I respect Imran and the work he does tremendously.

His organization recently ran an experiment. They created accounts on the site and listed the users as thirteen-year-old girls, which is the youngest age allowed by TikTok. Now, we know children younger than that get on TikTok, but within the experiment they played by TikTok's supposed rules, even if kids violate those rules all the time.

Imran's team watched to see what sorts of videos and content TikTok would show these thirteen-year-old girls.

What they found was incredibly disturbing. In less than three minutes, the TikTok algorithm—which is the program that tells the app what videos to show you—had started feeding content that promoted self-harm to these thirteen-year-old girls. Three minutes.

And kids don't look away or turn the phone off, because the content they get served is subtle, it's enticing, it's alluring.

The video might start with an aspirational image of a slim young woman in a beautiful outfit. So, a young girl starts watching it. Then, very quickly, it starts showing lines around the woman's waist saying, if you want a waist as small as mine, you need to have a 700-calorie diet. The longer you watch, the more similar messages it feeds you, because it "learns" you're vulnerable to those kinds of videos based on the amount of time you spent watching them and the number of times you continue to click or select that type of content when it is offered.

Another example of the danger pertains to self-harm content. You might be fed a picture of a razor blade with really emotional music. Then words start circling the razor blade, and they read, "I miss the touch of you on my skin." From there it starts feeding you more videos telling you it's good to cut yourself.

It is sick and bone-chilling stuff and I am confident the majority of parents have no idea that 1) their young daughter is off by herself watching this and that 2) this is the kind of content that is being served up to her.

So Imram and his team decided to push the experiment further. This time they gave one of their fake thirteen-year-olds a straightforward name, like Lauren or Sarah. The second one would be something like Lauren Lose Weight. This isn't as weird as it sounds; people can give themselves usernames on TikTok that describe their goals or the things they're into. The name signaled an area of interest. It signaled vulnerability. And the algorithm went about its ruthless work.

"Lauren Lose Weight" got twelve times the amount of self-harm content as the normal account and got three times the amount of overall harmful content as the normal account—which was already getting a ton of harmful content to begin with.

Why? Because The algorithm isn't a parent. It's not a friend. It doesn't care about you or your child or anyone else. It cares about your eyeballs; it cares about getting you addicted. It cares about keeping you watching, and clicking, and swiping. The algorithm is doing what any algorithm program is designed to do: whatever it takes to keep a user engaged longer and more actively. It is not concerned with whether that content is healthy or self-destructive. Its job is to keep people on the platform for as long as possible. It's trying to find any sort of indication as to the psychology of the user and bombarding them with videos that exploit that psychology.

> **The algorithm isn't a parent. It's not a friend. It doesn't care about you or your child or anyone else. It cares about your eyeballs; it cares about getting you addicted.**

This is why I say all the time that you aren't the only voice in your child's ear, so you had better be the *best* voice in that ear.

But here I'm sharing that story to make a different point.

Because if you're disgusted, scared, or pissed-off by this, I'm here to deliver some bad news.

The very same thing is being done to you.

You remember how back in the earlier days of Facebook, there was only one way to react to something you saw: a thumbs-up. They called it a "like." Something that made you smile, something that made you sad—same reaction, thumbs-up.

Then Facebook realized it was kind of weird that if somebody's dog died, the only way you could react was by giving them a "like," so they created other emojis you could react with—love, ha-ha, wow, sad, and angry. So far, so good. They were giving folks more and more accurate ways to react.

But then they did something that you didn't know. In fact, none of us knew it until a whistleblower came forward.[1] Facebook also has an algorithm, again a computer program, that decides what you see. And what Facebook did was start treating those emotional responses differently. In deciding to show you more of the material they thought you wanted to see, a "like" was worth one point. But all of a sudden, they decided that an angry response was worth five points. And so if something made you angry, all of a sudden you started seeing a lot more stuff that was very similar to the thing that made you angry in the first place.

Now you might think, "That's bad for my mental health, to have a platform I spent a lot of time on just feeding me things that make me angry," and you're right. But while it's bad for your mental health, it's also bad for another reason. Facebook found that the stuff that was making people angry was also likely to include misinformation!

So why would Facebook want to keep feeding you news that was making you angry, riddled with an uncommon amount of inaccurate information? I'll give you three guesses. If you guessed money, money, and—hmmm. Oh yeah, money—you got it!

They found that if you are emotionally invested, if you are emotionally upset, your level of engagement goes up. If you're looking at a box of kittens and it makes you feel good and puts a smile on your face, that may keep you clicking for a little while. But it doesn't get you on the edge of your chair, squeezing that mouse and clicking until your finger hurts. But if they're showing you things that upset you, things that you are just shaking your head about, then guess what? Before you know it, you are all in. More time and more clicks mean more exposure to ads and more money for them.

Lots of money.

The more time you spent on the site, the more you clicked and clicked and clicked and clicked—the more money they made.

They were the ones winning the offendedness sweepstakes. And they're not alone. Same with the cable news channels, Instagram and X (formerly known as Twitter), and everyone else who captures your attention by making you angry.

The most important thing to acknowledge is that what engaged you may have been discovered by accident. It may have been discovered by looking backward to see what people's viewing patterns were. But the practice of programming the site to feed you disturbing content wasn't an accident, despite their knowing that the material was mentally and emotionally upsetting. A conscious decision was made to choose profit over your well-being and that of your children.

A conscious decision was made to disregard whether or not you would experience increases in anxiety, depression, agitation, sleep disturbance, all the things that go along with emotional upheaval, in order to increase profits.

You lose, they win.

And boy are they winning. Because you are addicted. We are addicted. And most of us know it. Nearly half of us admit to being addicted to our smartphones.

Now, you can say, "I'm not addicted, I use it a reasonable amount."

And to that I would say, really? Then why are you checking it over 350 times a day?

That's right, the average American checks their smartphone 352 times a day.[2] About once every three minutes of every waking hour.

Why do you feel anxious if you've misplaced your phone?

Why do you actually check your phone *more* when it is silenced? (When phones are silenced, people have more fear of missing out and thus check their phone more frequently!)[3]

Needing the next fix. Experiencing symptoms of withdrawal. These are signs of addiction.

And that's just adults.

Children, whose brains aren't fully developed, may be even more susceptible. And two-thirds of children spend *four hours a day* or more on their smartphones.[4]

In 2023, America's surgeon general released a twenty-five-page advisory saying that there's not enough evidence to say that social media is "sufficiently safe" for children and teenagers.[5]

Let me translate that bit of mealymouthed government-speak:

phones and social media are dangerous, dangerous, dangerous. I would argue that any benefit from the ability to "find online communities" of like-minded young people is far outweighed by the risk of being exposed to—and addicted to—inappropriate and dangerous content.

The question is, what are you going to do about it? Are you willing to unplug? Or are you going to cave to "FOMO," the Fear of Missing Out? This is a very real syndrome. Fearing you are going to miss out on something relevant, something all the "cool kids" know about, is a very real syndrome.

So, let me reiterate some very real advice.

You are not the only voice in your child's ear, so you'd better be the *best* voice in that ear. Keep them off social media until they're thirteen.

When they're on the phone, set clear limits on both content and screen time.

They'll complain, for sure.

They'll agitate for more time and more freedom.

Protect now, and the respect will come later.

When I assert that the American family is under attack—as I do throughout this book—this is one of the specific things I'm talking about. It's not just that technological devices like smartphones, iPads, and laptops are competing for quality time between parents and children, which they are. It's that the devices are delivering content that has a negative impact on parents and children alike.

The devices are actually bringing toxicity into the family unit. That has been empirically proven by the internal studies of the social media companies themselves. If you didn't know it before, you know it now.

And we haven't even addressed exposure to online predators and other dangers.

The question is, what are you going to do about it? You cannot bury your head in the sand or you prove Russia right: we are "demoralized," we just let it happen.

POLL RESPONSES

How often do you read a news report or see a tweet that makes you angry?

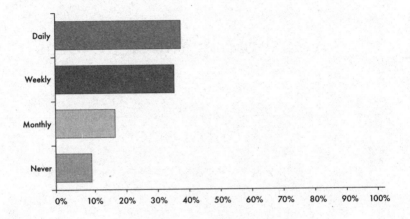

You're seeing things that upset you. What I'm setting forth in this chapter is that you need to consider the fact that that may not be coincidental, that may not be just happenstance. It may very well be that that's coming at you on purpose to engage you so you will stay on that site and allow them to feed you more and more that makes you upset. And the follow-up question you have to ask yourself is, "Am I okay with that? Am I okay with the fact that they are baiting me and then feeding me upsetting material so they can make money off of me?" And if that does upset you, you've got to consider unplugging.

CHAPTER 9

Censored by the Algorithm

POLL QUESTION

How often do you feel that you are being told the truth by the media?

- ☐ Always
- ☐ Very often
- ☐ Sometimes
- ☐ Never

While you're getting fed highly curated, highly filtered information, you aren't getting other information:

We're seeing revelation after revelation that the big social media platforms were censoring what information made its way to you, not based on your political leanings, but on *theirs*.

Now, I know the First Amendment doesn't guarantee free speech in private enterprise, and that nothing guarantees that everyone has an equal chance to be heard. But would you willingly let a big company decide for you what you hear and see and what you don't hear and see?

Because that's what you're doing right now. As a result, someone is deciding that the story you get isn't the whole story; the story you get might be the story they want you to see and not the one they don't want you to see. Sometimes it's the story that will upset you enough that it will keep you engaged. Sometimes it's the golden ticket and it's both! The real problem is that someone who is making the decision is *not* you.

Doesn't that make you wonder who that someone is, what their agenda is, and why it is hidden? It certainly makes me curious.

People use social media platforms for different reasons, such as to connect with others and get what they mistakenly think is peer validation (or confuse as real socialization). But, while they are on those platforms, algorithms—specifically, machine-learning algorithms—collect all kinds of data on their activities.

This data is used to understand users' preferences, accurately target ads, and curate personalized content. Although the aforementioned *might be* fine and even, in some ways, helpful in serving up what users want, problems arise when algorithms are manipulated or programmed to influence users' actions or feelings *deliberately*, to comport to the political views of someone at the company that owns the platform.

Think about that: the algorithm is programmed to influence what you do or what you feel and they are doing it on purpose, without you being aware.

Even more troubling is when these algorithms infringe on users' fundamental rights to free expression, association, and equal treatment.

Specifically, on social media platforms, such as Facebook, X (formerly known as Twitter), and Instagram, we discussed the fact that the algorithm is geared, first and foremost, to keep you clicking.

However, they also create an "echo chamber" effect, where you only see content that confirms your beliefs, isolating you from differing points of view. Think MSNBC versus Fox News.

I firmly believe that this can undermine your freedom of thought, conscience, and communication. You may never be confronted with information that makes you say, "Wow! I never thought of it that way."

And if you live your life never having been confronted with a different point of view, you lose perspective. You lose the ability to see, understand, or empathize with a differing point of view.

You may think you're getting served what you want. And the platforms may think you're getting served what they think you need. But you quickly realize that the only person who doesn't have a say in what you get served . . . is you.

> **You may think you're getting served what you want. And the platforms may think you're getting served what they think you need. But you quickly realize that the only person who doesn't have a say in what you get served . . . is you.**

Just as an algorithm takes any predilections and predispositions you have and compounds them by serving you what it thinks you want, it also compounds our societal predilections toward racism. There's actually a term for this: *algorithmic bias.*

This occurs when the algorithm incorporates prejudices along racial, gender, and other lines into a system of what it selects to share with you. That can happen by either promoting or burying content, discriminating, and limiting the reach of specific groups or topics. Such biased algorithms can erode freedoms by disproportionately pushing certain political stories. It can actually affect democratic processes.

It does this by making it challenging for people or ideas that are not currently "popular" to gain traction because they are suppressed, or, conversely, it can push nonmainstream ideas into the mainstream based on what whoever controls the algorithm wants to be seen. Additionally, individuals and topics can be "blacklisted" or "shadow banned"—pushed out of view or silenced altogether. Sometimes this is done as a thoughtful decision by a "content moderation team"—to keep dangerous misinformation or disinformation at bay. But it can also be done at the request of a powerful individual—like a business or political leader.

You see how this can pose a grave threat to free speech and participation in the democratic process. Again, none of this is illegal in any way. There are no First Amendment requirements for private business. The problem is that democracy is supposed to operate like a "town square"—where all ideas are heard and judged. The ways social media platforms operate today are like "town squares" where people go to talk about what's on their minds. In fact, some of them even refer to themselves as such.

Except they aren't, because we're now living in a world in which the First Amendment limits government interference in private speech but not the behavior of private entities. Social media companies can do what government can't: they can suppress views that are protected under the First Amendment.

The biggest concern is that it's all hidden; it's all invisible to you and me. In 2004, the former Soviet dissident and human rights activist Natan Sharansky wrote a book called *The Case for Democracy*. In it, Sharansky created what he called the "town square test." The way to know if you're living in a fear society, he wrote, is "if a person cannot walk into the middle of the town square and express his or her views without the fear of arrest, imprisonment, or physical harm. . . ."[1]

By that definition, we're not living in a "fear society"—at least not yet. In a fear society, in a real town square, when a person is getting silenced, you actually see them getting attacked, or muzzled, or arrested, or dragged away.

In an algorithmic censorship society—which I fear we're moving toward—you don't see anything. You don't hear the dissenting or unpopular voice. You don't hear the new or different idea. You never knew they even existed to begin with.

One thing I learned during my time working with juries in the litigation arena is that a strong component of human nature is that people make decisions based on what they see and hear, not on what they don't see and hear.

It may sound obvious: of course you make a decision on what you see and not on what you don't. But it's an important insight. You can imply or suggest that there's another idea out there, that there's a different way of looking at something, a different interpretation. I watched lawyers do it hundreds of times. It's not a winning strategy, because no matter how strongly someone implies that there is more to the story, people don't respond to it unless they are actually told the story.

And often, because of someone else's decision, you aren't getting the whole story. As this selective censorship has come to light in the last few years, we have learned who the mysterious "wizards" behind the curtain are. Who it is that has been making the decisions about what you and I see in our "feeds" on social media. We have learned that the heads of these major platforms, like Facebook and their team of executives, have been meeting and reviewing documents and stories with representatives of the FBI and other officials to decide what we get to see.

Now, I don't happen to agree on a lot of social or cultural issues with these individuals, so I feel really jerked around. However, even if I did agree with their positions on the social and cultural issues, I wouldn't feel any less so. Why? Because I don't like people sneaking around my back and manipulating what I see and hear. I don't like being stuck in a bubble and only hearing one side of a story, issue, or situation whether I agree with it or not.

Either way, now that I know what I know, I wouldn't trust any of them in an outhouse with a muzzle on.

POLL RESPONSE

How often do you feel you are being told the truth by the media?

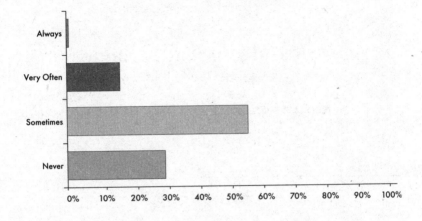

CHAPTER 10

Avoid Logical Fallacies

Presentism, Confirmation Bias, and Positive Bias

POLL QUESTION

Have you been judged or criticized in your current life for something you may have done many years ago when the rules and expectations were different?

☐ Yes

☐ No

As we work to deprogram ourselves, we need to recognize that there are a lot more ways to get you outraged and pull your strings that are subtler than an outright lie, and I want you to be on guard against them.

Consider something called *presentism*. This is where we apply today's rules and values to yesterday's situations. Said another way, it is the interpretation of past events in the light of present-day attitudes, rather than in the light of their own historical context.

Times change, mores and folkways change, rules and laws change, but presentists apply the standards of today to the conduct of yesteryear. To follow their logic, people one or two hundred years ago were somehow supposed to know that a couple of centuries in the future, things would be different and therefore they had to behave according to the standards of the future.

Absolutely absurd.

To embrace that mindset, you have to be so arrogant and narcissistic as to think that if you were alive two hundred years ago you would have been so enlightened and so ahead of your time that you would have behaved differently than everyone else around you.

If we can't keep up with the mores and folkways of our own time, how can we expect someone to live according to those two hundred years in the future?!

But some people, since they weren't alive two hundred years ago, have become the self-appointed "presentism police," performing citizen's arrests on people from yesteryear and judging them by today's standards.

Here's a more current example: Imagine you drive a certain road to work every day for a year and the speed limit is 55, which you abide by religiously. One day the town decides to change the speed limit to 40. Presentism would result in the town giving you a *retroactive* ticket for thousands of dollars because you've been going 15 over the *new* speed limit *before it was the new speed limit*! Even though you were obeying the speed limit at the time, you are now being ticketed *retroactively* and fined for failing to obey the new standard before it was even a standard. I know what you're thinking; that would never stand up in a court of law. You are 100 percent correct. But that sort of accusation can *and does* win in the court of public opinion, especially when people don't know all the facts.

Sounds kind of silly, but we've seen presentism in practice in all sorts of places. Earlier in my career, I represented a company that was being sued for billions of dollars for polluting a river. The problem was that there was no law against them doing what they were doing at the time when they were doing it. What's more, at the time, nobody knew the chemicals they were disposing of were even pollutants. No one had a clue they were dangerous. They were disposing of wastewater in a totally acceptable and approved manner for that day and time. So, now that we know more, we absolutely should all work together to clean it up, but to say that the company was a "bad actor" is presentism.

Or, look more recently. Back in 2021, the New York City Council made a unanimous decision. It wasn't about crime or poverty. It was about removing a statue of Thomas Jefferson that had stood in the city council chambers for over one hundred years.[1]

As one council member said, Jefferson had to go because he "embodied some of the most shameful parts of our country's long and nuanced history."

Indeed, he did. He owned slaves, as was common practice at the time. Common but absolutely terrible. At the time, however, it was not unlawful. Should it have been? Absolutely. Was it a stain on our history? Without question. But he also did a lot of great things.

And the statue was there to honor the fact that *he wrote the Declaration of Independence*, perhaps the greatest statement of human freedom in the history of the world. In fact, the most proslavery people in America at the time hated him for that, because they knew he had planted the seeds of future freedom. Jefferson may have been one of the most forward-thinking leaders in the history of the world, but he wasn't forward-thinking enough for the New York City Council 250 years later.

Presentism says that we can't honor Jefferson because the rules have changed between his time and ours. I submit to you what I believe is a more reasonable approach: it's better to keep the statue and give our elected officials a daily reminder of how complicated human beings are, and how the real tragedy isn't falling short of grand aspirations; it's in not having any grand aspirations at all.

A few pages ago, I said that the scary thing that's happening today is that we're big-brothering *each other*, that it's not the government doing it. Someone works hard and does a good job and is picked for a great accolade. The "presentism police" swing into action and go back and find some idiotic tweet he or she posted as a *teenager*, and the next thing you see, hear, and read is "Gotcha!" Does a decades-old tweet reflect who they are? Does it make people around them unsafe? Does it mean that they are a racist or bigot or homophobe? In most cases, the answer is clearly no.

But what is the value of someone's reputation, career, and psyche when you stack it up against the free publicity that can be gained from finding that old tweet and tearing someone down? I think people say things when they're young that don't truly reflect who they are. I think people grow and change with the times. Not every past transgression is worthy of present-day cancellation. Heck, most of those past transgressions weren't even transgressions at the time. But who cares who they really are and how they really feel as long as you get a few headlines for the cause, right? I think personal and societal evolution does matter, and I'm betting you do too. I'm also betting, and I'm certainly hoping, that you have decided along with me that enough is enough and too much is too much.

I will point out again, this is not the government stepping in and dropping the hammer on our rights; this is us doing it to each other. Maybe it bothers you and maybe it doesn't, but I'll bet that if and when the day comes that you find yourself in the crosshairs of the mob, when it's your turn and they come after you, your level of compassion will change.

It's too bad that we have to personally experience certain things to really activate and mobilize our energy and compassion. But it's also human nature. Sometimes our compassion is limited to our own experience. How often do we see someone lose a loved one to a drunk driver and then become a crusader to stop drunk driving?

Or we lose someone to a terrible disease and immediately start a foundation to help fight that disease?

Don't get me wrong, it's great that that happens at all for whatever reason. I just pray that we broaden our compassion beyond our own experience.

When we are big-brothering *ourselves* (as Yuri, the former KGB spy whom we met in chapter 7, pointed out), we fall prey to *confirmation bias*—which is our tendency to seek out and only process data that confirms what we already believe, and *self-referential reasoning*, which is when we only hear what we want to hear.

Say just for argument's sake that you think all police are jack-booted, heavy-handed, trigger-happy racists. Every story you see about a police-involved shooting or police brutality is going to support that belief, regardless of the facts of the specific situation. And remember, as I showed you a couple of pages ago, the minute you express anger about something a police officer did, every social media platform is going to start feeding you information that makes you angrier and angrier. That algorithm is going to feed you that kind of story like meat to a hungry bear. And when that's all you see your belief system is going to get deeper and narrower.

> When we are big-brothering *ourselves*, we fall prey to *confirmation bias*—which is our tendency to seek out and only process data that confirms what we already believe, and *self-referential reasoning*, which is when we only hear what we want to hear.

Now say you have a Blue Lives Matter flag flying on your house, and you believe that police are the most dedicated public servants there are, doing a difficult job to the best of their abilities, walking out of the house each day knowing there's a chance they won't come home—something that happens hundreds of times a year.[2] And you read every story you see about a police officer being ambushed or killed or even disrespected, which means you're going to keep seeing more of those stories.

If you're in the "all cops are bad" school of thought, suppose I bring you information that says that there are about 800,000 police officers in this country, and the vast majority of them have never fired their service weapon on the job, not once.[3] And that most who do fire their weapon have never fired it before—meaning they were in some situation where it seemed absolutely necessary. That information won't matter to you, you simply won't hear it, because it runs counter to your confirmation bias. Research tells us that not only will it not change your belief, but it may actually deepen your belief even though it runs empirically counter to what you believe.

If you're in the Blue Lives Matter school, and I show you data that says that actually there are some police officers who are much more likely to fire their weapons and kill innocent people—they're white military veterans who are policing big cities, we know who they are, we can screen out most bad cops before they ever hit the streets. Or that you, the taxpayer, are paying a share of the billions—yes, billions—of settlement money that's paid out as a result of police misconduct, you don't want to hear that either.[4]

Look, I don't want to diminish the human impact of this issue. I have talked to the widows and widowers of fallen officers. I have a personal relationship with Ahmaud Arbery's parents. I have a personal relationship with George Floyd's mother. I've seen their pain. You've probably seen me sit with those families and interview them. And the problem is that solutions never lie at one end or the other. The solution isn't defunding the police. And the solution isn't denying that there are some folks out there who are dangerously badge-heavy and trigger-happy.

Retraining law enforcement officers is great, to a degree. It is already happening across America in police departments large and small. The impact, of course, depends on several factors, including the quality and the objective of the training. It is also important to monitor where officers are mentally, emotionally, and in terms of attitude.

They are human beings who have stressful and occasionally traumatic jobs, and when they go home, they are subject to the pressures of life just like everyone else.

What you absolutely do not want to do is to train officers to try to wear too many hats in what can prove to be very dangerous situations. It is true that the majority of day-to-day police work is misdemeanor-level situations. But every interaction with the public has the potential to become difficult.

Police officers are charged with enforcing the law. They don't make the laws; they aren't there to empathize with why someone might be breaking the law.

They are there to suppress criminal behavior, get the situation under control, and protect everyone involved as quickly and safely as humanly possible. An unfortunate reality of the job is that they often meet members of the public when those people are in anything other than their finest hour, when they are distressed or distraught and sometimes at the end of their range of coping skills. We want our police suppressing potentially dangerous behavior before it deteriorates into violent or lethal behavior.

You do not want them doing therapy or analysis on the scene; you want calm, unbiased efficiency.

Everyone can always do better. Police officers are no exception, and should be held to the highest standards. If and when they fail to meet those standards, if they abuse the power invested in them when they are given a badge and a gun, they should be taken off the street and held accountable.

But I need to point out that there are not enough hours in their busy days to adequately train them to make solid psychological judgments about the potential danger of an individual at the spur of the moment.

For their survival and maybe yours, they need to assume that all individuals they are called to intervene with are potentially dangerous until they are under control and can be safely interacted with. It is their job to suppress potentially dangerous behavior safely and efficiently.

Training officers to effectively defuse situations to reduce the likelihood of injury is a great goal. But the officer's job is to get an alleged perpetrator under control to a point that a properly trained counselor or social worker on the team can safely intervene. That is the proper division of labor.

This might well involve redirecting money for police departments, but it certainly doesn't suggest reducing money for police departments. These men and women are putting themselves in harm's way every single day, in order to keep the rest of us safe. I, for one, appreciate that fact and I try to never pass a uniformed officer on the sidewalk without stopping, shaking his or her hand, and thanking them for the work they do. I invite you to do the same.

This reality is like a lot of other challenges we face in our society today. Again, it is about identifying the problem and finding a solution (as I discuss in Principle #2), and confirmation bias makes that a lot harder.

Confirmation bias and self-referential reasoning lead you to stop becoming a consumer of information and turn you into an advocate for your worldview. They allow us to live in a world where we only hear what we want to hear.

All of this is supercharged by something our brain does called *automatic thinking*. We start filling in all sorts of blanks without even knowing it—it's the brain running on autopilot, using shortcuts to speed up mental processes to get us to an answer, a conclusion, or a decision. The problem with automatic thinking is that it depends on things you've seen or learned before. If one of your coworkers screwed up once, and you see that there's another screwup, your brain is more likely to assume that that coworker was involved. Automatic thinking sometimes gets you to the right answer, but it can also reinforce the wrong answers too.

Positive Bias

There was a period of several years where, as part of my work, I debriefed thousands and thousands of mock and real jurors a year, as I'll explain below. I was trying to understand what information moved them, what made one witness believable and another look like a liar. And those witnesses taught me something so obvious that it's actually profound.

We believe who we like.

We like who likes us.

So, we believe who likes us.

Jurors were more likely to believe lawyers and witnesses whom they liked. They were more likely to believe lawyers and witnesses who provided cues to them that they liked them—respecting their intelligence and dedication, smiling at them—what we call "minimal encouragers."

Salespeople, of course, have figured this out already. Their living depends on it. How many times have you heard a car salesman say, "I don't usually do this, but I *like* you, so let me see what I can make work"? You like them because they like the cut of your jib!

Think of yourself at a party with a group of people you don't know. You have a nice evening, you tell some stories, you share some laughs. When you're home later that night, reflecting on the evening, who did you meet that you liked? Without realizing it, you probably liked the person who laughed at your joke, who nodded along (there are those "minimal encouragers" again) at your story, or who asked you questions about it. You liked the person who liked you, the person who was a good audience and made you feel welcome, accepted, and interesting.

We often think of the word *bias* as negative. But this is just one of several positive "biases." And a positive bias is as likely to get someone in trouble as a negative bias. If a friend comes to you and asks you

to do something that you suspect might be legally or ethically bor-
derline, you're more likely to do it. You want to help the person who
likes you.

Another positive bias is the bias toward the highly credentialed.
Why does your doctor have all of those diplomas on the walls—even
if you can't read half of them because they're in Latin? Because you're
going to feel a lot better about being cut open by someone who is
highly credentialed. In his autobiography, Michael Eisner, who was
an iconic CEO of the Walt Disney Company at the time, talks about
being at a conference and having upper-arm pain and shortness of
breath. He needed heart surgery. As they were about to perform the
operation, he called his wife over to ask about the doctor who was
scheduled to do his surgery. "Where was this guy trained?" he asked.
In the book, he writes, "She knew I was hoping to hear Harvard or
Yale. 'Tijuana,' she replied, with a straight face."[5] Why is this story
funny? Because this big-swinging-you-know-what CEO wanted to
know that he was under the care of the best; he had a positive bias
toward the highly credentialed.

We also have a bias toward exclusivity. Groucho Marx once said,
"I don't want to belong to any club that would accept me as one of
its members." It's funny because we all want to be part of something
more exclusive than we think we belong to.

Bernie Madoff ran the largest Ponzi scheme in history—a $64 bil-
lion scheme that allowed him to steal about $18 billion from his "inves-
tors." How was he able to get so many investors to flock to his fraud?
Exclusivity bias. He was the club you had to know someone to get into.
Listen to Burt Ross, the former mayor of Fort Lee, New Jersey. He sent
Madoff $2 million. He described getting into Madoff's fund like get-
ting into Harvard. "It took pull. My friend had to call somebody . . .
and he reached Madoff in Europe. And I got papal dispensation. This
is part of the scam . . . you have to understand, this was a genius. The
harder it was to get in, the more you wanted to get in."[6]

The point is to check yourself for biases in either positive or negative directions. Test your beliefs. Be honest with yourself about how you feel and why. Winners deal with the truth, the facts, the data. Not just what is being pushed on them.

POLL RESPONSE

Have you been judged or criticized in your current life for something you may have done many years ago when the rules and expectations were different?

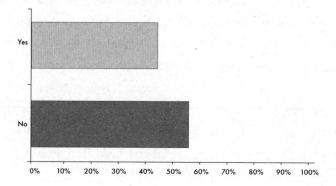

I get how unfair this is. The rules change across time. And to hold you to today's standards for yesterday's behavior is just not right. If you have been judged that way, you are not alone. Over half the people in the sample share that experience with you, and for the over half of you that haven't, I hope that remains to be the case. And hopefully after reading what I have had to say in this book, when it does come knocking on your door you'll know how to fight back.

CHAPTER 11

Are You Open to Changing Your Mind?

POLL QUESTION

Once you have made up your mind about something of importance, how likely are you to revisit the decision and actually
change your mind and adopt a new position?

- ☐ Always
- ☐ Very often
- ☐ Sometimes
- ☐ Never

One of the things we see in psychology is that it's very difficult—
almost painful—to open up our minds to new information, to
embrace a new way of thinking.

Early in my career, I started a company called Courtroom Sciences
Inc. (CSI), a trial sciences company. Our job was to help our clients
prepare for trial by, among other things, helping lawyers understand
how juries would react to what they were hearing in the courtroom.
In fact, the only reason you've ever heard of me is because of CSI.

That's because one of the defendants we helped was Oprah Winfrey. That's how I came to know Oprah, and how you got to know me.

Now, in a trial, the prosecution speaks first. They're the ones bringing the case, and so they have the burden of proof. Speaking first gives them an advantage. They start with a jury that's a totally blank canvas, and the prosecution gets to paint a picture of the case.

I describe it this way. A jury is sitting there at the beach, on the beach blanket, and the prosecution starts walking them across the burning-hot sand to get their feet to the cool water. In this example, the cool water is a clear understanding of the case, and a decision as to who is at fault. The hot burning sand is the pain of conflict. People hate to be in conflict. They want to get out of that uncomfortable position as quickly as they possibly can. And the prosecution, in that opening statement, takes them either almost all the way there or all the way there. As I have often said, your story is going to go a lot better when you are the only one telling it. The jury wants to hear something—anything—that lets them get their feet off the hot sand and in the cool water. It is just human nature.

Then the defense has to get up and say: Not so fast. Instead of getting all the way to that cool water, or even standing comfortably in it, I want you to turn around and walk back across the hot sand and sit back down on the beach blanket. It's not easy. And for the jury, it's almost that painful. They were in the pain of conflict and the plaintiff or prosecutor got them out of it. Now you're wanting them to reopen the issue and get back into that conflict situation again, and trust me, that's a tough sale.

That's what it's like to open up your mind to new information, to a new way of seeing the world, perhaps even to seeing the truth. I fully realize I may be putting you into a conflict situation in your own mind. I may be creating a high degree of dissonance. But "we" cannot remain silent any longer. As uncomfortable as it may be to consider, if we resolve to take this country back, you're going to have to open your mind to reexamining some things that you may have just been letting slide. Our country and your future happiness, health, and security could very well be at stake.

Not only are we losing our curiosity, but we're punishing people who push us to be curious, who want us to walk on the hot sand.

For example, I'm acquainted with a woman named Bari Weiss, who was an editor at the *New York Times*, responsible for the opinion pages. Since opinion isn't news, she set out to bring different voices to the newspaper—centrists and conservatives, mainly.

For this transgression against curiosity and confirmation bias, for daring to try to break down people's bubbles and get them to hear an opinion that was different than their own, an opinion that, God forbid, might make them uncomfortable, she was attacked, vilified, and threatened to the point where she had no choice but to resign.

In her resignation letter, she said something that is a warning to us all: "a new consensus has emerged . . . that truth isn't a process of collective discovery, but an orthodoxy already known to an enlightened few whose job is to inform everyone else."

When someone claims they have a monopoly on truth, it's a pretty safe bet they don't. And if you give yourself over to their view of the world—without questioning, without thinking, without investigating—you're giving up one of the things that make America great. Self-determination.

To fully understand the forces that are at work on you, and how you react to them, it helps to have a better understanding *of you.*

Starting in the mid-1900s, researchers began studying the words people use to describe themselves and others. Their idea was that humans are really good at noticing differences between one another. And when we notice a difference enough times, we give it a word. For example, over years and years, humans noticed that some people are very cooperative, and they try to make others feel more comfortable, and we come up with a word like *agreeable*. Or that some people keep to themselves a lot and seem to live in a world of ideas—and we create the word *introverted* to describe them.

In the 1970s, researchers surveyed thousands of people and found that most descriptions clustered around five main personality traits. These traits are:[1]

- ➤ Openness

- ➤ Conscientiousness

- ➤ Extroversion

- ➤ Agreeableness

- ➤ Neuroticism

As a result, this came to be called the "OCEAN" test. And until recently, it was considered the gold standard in personality testing.

At around that time, two young graduate students in Canada—Michael Ashton and Kibeom Lee—conducted a research study where they asked Korean students about their personalities, using Korean personality trait terms. As they analyzed their findings, they realized there were actually **six main characteristics**.

Then they checked results from research studies in Italian, German, Hungarian, Dutch, and other languages, and they found the same six. They saw the same results in a new study in the English language—results different in some ways from the OCEAN findings.

For example, some of the traits that had fallen into the category of agreeableness in the OCEAN test actually were their own category—which Ashton and Lee describe as honesty/humility. Several other traits became a little more focused as well. So you end up with:

- ➤ **Honesty-Humility.** This includes measures of characteristics like fairness, sincerity, modesty, and lack of greed.

- ➤ **Emotionality.** Here we're talking about being emotionally

sensitive—traits like anxiety, fearfulness, dependence, and
sentimentality.

➤ **Extraversion.** This involves traits like self-esteem, boldness, sociability, and liveliness.

➤ **Agreeableness.** This is about characteristics like forgiveness, gentleness, flexibility, and patience.

➤ **Conscientiousness.** This gets at being conscientious with
tasks—traits like organization, diligence, perfectionism,
and prudence.

➤ **Openness to Experience.** This looks at how much you
appreciate art and culture, how curious you are, how creative you are, and how original or conventional you are.

It's really amazing when you think about it. Different cultures,
using different languages, across different eras still found words clus-
tering around the same handful of personality traits.

Professors Ashton and Lee (they got their doctorates in the
meantime and began teaching) called this modified test HEXACO,
and it is fast becoming one of the gold standards in self-administered
personality testing. This isn't some quiz you'd see in a fashion magazine. It's a real, scientifically backed, widely accepted way of understanding a bit more about your personality traits. Understand, it is
not designed to find or differentiate mental disorders, and no such
label will be generated by the test. It is not looking for mental illness
or any pathology.

Everyone has these global traits to a greater or lesser degree, and
being at a high percentile is not necessarily better than being at a
low percentile on a given trait. So, no one can do "better" or "worse"
than anyone else, only different.

And that's why I think it will be useful and informative for *you* to
take the HEXACO test.

Here's what you can expect. It's one hundred questions, and it will take about twenty minutes.

A couple of things to note before you jump in:

➤ Sometimes your results don't match your own perceptions. That's okay. That's how you learn about yourself. Sometimes it can be useful to ask a friend or loved one to take the test and answer questions as they see them applying to you. So, they would respond in the way they perceive you to be. That way you can see if your view of yourself matches up with someone else's view of you, and then you can do the same for them.

➤ The test won't just ask you: Are you open? That doesn't really work. It asks questions that are not so obvious but have, across thousands and thousands of people, been shown to reveal to what degree you're open to new experiences or ideas. The questions get you to reveal a "behavioral tendency" that connects with one of the traits.

➤ A "higher" score isn't better or worse. There's no one ideal level of a personality trait.

➤ Your results will be anonymous. No one but you will see them unless you choose to share them. That means it is in your best interest to answer as openly, honestly, and candidly as you possibly can. Don't try to "outthink the test" because you want the feedback you get to be as valid as possible.*

Once you've taken the test, you'll see your results in a graph. You'll receive a percentile score and a "scale score" for each of the six major

---

* To get your percentile scores, your results will be combined with other people's results. However, they will remain anonymous, and used only for academic research.

personality traits. For example, your "extraversion" score may be a 5.5 and your "sociability percentile" may be 65 percent. The scores are calculated so that 5 is always average. And the percentile scores tell you what percent of people test below that percentile. So, a 5.5 and a 65 percent says: you demonstrate and experience a little more of the characteristics associated with the extraversion trait (which include boldness, sociability, social self-esteem, and liveliness) than average, and 65 percent of people who have taken the test before you and are anonymously in the database answered the same questions in a way that they scored as experiencing less of those characteristics than you. That's all a way of saying that this survey is about *insight*. It's a window into your basic disposition.

Again, it's not a diagnostic tool.

It's not a "prophecy" about your future. But you can use it to begin to adjust some of your attitudes and behaviors.

Let's find out where we're starting from:

If this code isn't working, you can also go to hexaco.org and click on "Take the HEXACO-PI-R." (PI-R stands for "Personality Inventory, Revised.")

POLL RESPONSE

Once you have made up your mind about something of importance, how likely are you to revisit that decision and actually change your mind and adopt a new position?

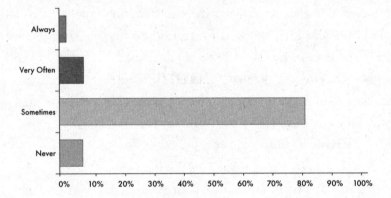

Now, you may be thinking, didn't I already answer this question back in chapter 7? Not exactly. That question asked if you'd revisit an opinion and seek out new information. This question is about actually changing your position. That's a harder—and rarer—thing to do.

CHAPTER 12

The Dangerous Temptation
of Victimhood

POLL QUESTION

Excluding being the victim of an actual crime, how many times in your life have you felt that someone's words and actions made you feel like your rights or feelings or humanity were actively attacked?

- ☐ More than ten times
- ☐ Five to ten times
- ☐ Between one and five times
- ☐ Never

If you answered affirmatively to the preceding question, how long did it take you to move past that initial feeling of injustice?

- ☐ A week or less
- ☐ A month
- ☐ A year
- ☐ I still haven't gotten over it

Every single one of us has a personal truth—something we believe about ourselves when nobody else is watching and we are just talking to ourselves about who we really believe we are. Our personal truth is what we really say to ourselves when our social mask is off.

I've spoken honestly about growing up with my own damaged personal truth.

Like a lot of folks, I grew up on the cusp between poverty and the lower class.

Education: never a family focus.

Alcoholic father: certainly not ideal.

Chaos and violence in the family: not good.

Sometimes it was better living on the streets, and so I did.

Other times it was a crummy apartment with no electricity or heat. No transportation. No "silver spoon" in my mouth at birth. Sometimes no spoon at all.

When I was young, I'd make the mistake a lot of us make—comparing my personal truth to someone else's social mask. I'd go to school and the kid sitting next to me would have freshly combed hair, pressed shirt and pants, and I'd think: "That's a buttoned-up kid, he's got a buttoned-up life."

Meanwhile, at my house that morning, we didn't know where the car was.

No way I could not compare and think, "I'm a second-class citizen."

Of course, comparing your personal truth to someone else's social mask is like comparing apples and oranges. You don't know their life, their story. I didn't know the life of that kid sitting next to me.

Unless we've really had a chance to sit and talk together, I also don't know yours.

But there is something I can say with confidence about your life: *you are not a victim.*

Earlier in this book, I talked about how the language police have become so overzealous. Like how you can't say that someone is "homeless" or was a "slave" because that somehow denies that they are first and foremost a person. That's where we get "enslaved person" or "person experiencing homelessness." Although, as a person who experienced homelessness, it didn't much matter to me if you said I was homeless or "a person experiencing homelessness." Neither term put a roof over my head. I was the one who had to do that.

But I'm going to turn the language police's tactics on them here. Because if we can't use descriptors like *homeless* or *slave*, I've got one more we should throw on the fire: *victim*.

You are not a victim. You may have had a run of bad luck or bad events. You may have had something tragic happen to you. You may have experienced a trauma. You may have a damaged personal truth, as I'll discuss in a moment. But you are not a victim. You only become a victim when you embrace a victimhood mindset—when you develop a tendency for interpersonal victimhood.

I want you to take a moment and pull out a pencil and rate on a 1–5 scale, with 1 being "not me at all" and 5 being "this is so me," how much you agree with each of these statements.[1]

It is important to me that people who hurt me acknowledge that an injustice has been done to me.
1—not me at all 2 3 4 5—this is so me

I think I am much more conscientious and moral in my relations with other people compared to their treatment of me.
1—not me at all 2 3 4 5—this is so me

When people who are close to me feel hurt by my actions, it is very important for me to clarify that justice is on my side.
1—not me at all 2 3 4 5—this is so me

It is very hard for me to stop thinking about the injustice others have done to me.
1—not me at all   2 3 4 5—this is so me

If you scored high (4 or 5) on all of these items, you may have what psychologists have identified as a "tendency for interpersonal victimhood."

(This quiz is adapted from one that appeared in *Scientific American*.)

My guess is that as you went through these questions, something or someone immediately came to mind. On question one, maybe you thought of someone who has been hounding you for an apology for something you can't even remember doing. Maybe they want you to acknowledge how hurtful it was that you didn't show up at their party. Maybe you remember confronting someone about a way in which they wronged you.

On question two, maybe you know someone who always sounds like a martyr, talking about how much better they have been to others than others have been to them. How they get no respect.

On question three, how many times have you seen someone explain their actions by citing justice? Someone cuts another person off in traffic claiming they have the right of way (as if anyone ever knows exactly who has the right of way), or someone steals something from a store because "this store has been stealing from me forever."

On question four, how often have you encountered someone who can't stop talking about how the server at the restaurant was rude to them, or how their boss never gives them credit? In my family, we jokingly called it Irish Alzheimer's—you forget everything but the slights.

But it also has a real title: Tendency for Interpersonal Victimhood (TIV). Put another way, it's a victimhood mindset.

And that tendency is defined by four traits that ultimately aren't good for you or society.

1. Need for Recognition

Victims aren't in charge of their lives, their stories, or their outcomes. People who see themselves as victims tend to deal with their grievances by calling them out, and then asking third parties to address the perceived injustice. To get a third party to act, victims call attention to themselves and their "plight."

2. Moral Elitism

Because a victim has come out on the losing end of some conflict, real or perceived, victims adopt an attitude of moral superiority. They see themselves as "better" than their victimizers. Which leads to a . . .

3. Lack of Empathy

If you feel like you're always being wronged, you are more likely to feel "owed" by society. That's entitlement, and if you walk through the world feeling entitled to things, you're less likely to care about how your actions affect others.

4. Rumination

Victims ruminate, or obsess, over their status, over the slights they've received. A victim is so busy looking backward that it's nearly impossible for them to move forward. Put another way, victims are miserable. They enjoy being miserable. I'll say it again: misery is not a strategy. At some point you stop being a victim, and you start being a *volunteer*.

Victimhood is a dangerous temptation.

You Are the Only One Who Sees Your Scar

In the late 1980s, Dr. Robert Kleck, a professor in the Department of Psychological and Brain Sciences at Dartmouth College, did an experiment. He had researchers use costume makeup to paint a scar on the faces of several women. The experiment involved these women, newly "scarred," having a face-to-face conversation with another person. But there was a catch. Before they left the room with their scar, the researchers said, "Hold on a second, I need to put some powder on your scar to prevent it from smearing." But they didn't add powder—they *erased* the scar entirely. The women didn't know it, but there was no longer any scar. They then went and had the conversation with a stranger and were asked to report on it. The women said that the stranger had stared at the scar and made them uncomfortable, that the stranger had been ruder to them than they otherwise would have been.[2]

That's a victimhood mentality. Victimhood tells you that you have a scar that everyone is staring at. You have a feature that makes you *less than* in some way. That you're seen differently. That you're being discriminated against, even when you aren't.

But when someone has embraced "victimhood culture," they bully others into embracing their story and accepting their ideologies. After all, it's not enough to say, "I'm a victim." Victimhood culture requires others believing it as well. "Victim" is no longer something passing that happened to you that you've worked to overcome—a personal tragedy, a natural disaster. It's now an integral part of your identity.

Zero Victim Thinking

A friend of mine and someone I respect very much, Pastor James Ward, says that a victim mentality is like being in a maximum-security prison with no walls. You're the only person keeping yourself there.

I recently had a conversation with Pastor Ward, who leads Insight Church, outside of Chicago. Pastor Ward also wrote a powerful book called *Zero Victim: Overcoming Injustice with a New Attitude*.

In it, Pastor Ward shared his personal story. Growing up in Tuscaloosa, Alabama, as a young man Pastor Ward was bused to school on the north side of town, the "white" side of town. It was the first time he ever saw a white student. He had a teacher who, whenever a student did well, put their names up on the board. And Pastor Ward started to see his name on the board quite a bit. All of a sudden, he realized: he wasn't inferior, nobody was holding him down, or holding him back. Yes, there may have been others in that class or in that town who were racist, who thought he was inferior, who would close a door to him. But, as he said, "when you know your identity, you cannot possibly be convinced that you are something or someone other than who you know you are."

Part of why I think Pastor Ward has it right is that he doesn't deny that real victimization exists. Terrible things do happen to people. People are discriminated against in all kinds of ways. In fact, he argues that it's almost inevitable. But victim*hood* is optional. A victim mentality exists when we allow the unfortunate circumstances of life to systematically control and dictate our quality of life.

Pastor Ward preaches a type of resilience he calls "zero victim" thinking, and I love the analogy he uses to describe it. Imagine the biggest, scariest baseball pitcher you know. They can throw a rock-hard fastball 100 miles an hour. Now, if you're just standing there and the pitch comes straight at you, it can hurt you. It can kill you. But if you have the right protective equipment, you're in the proper stance, and you stretch out a gloved hand in anticipation, then you can catch that pitch all day long. All of a sudden, what to one person (a victim) could be life-threatening becomes (to the catcher) a sport. Our national pastime. "The pitches are going to come. The victimization is going to come. . . . The world is a hostile place. The way that we prepare and precondition our minds to deal with those things determine whether or not they have effect on us."

If you think you can't get ahead, you have no incentive to try to get ahead. Again, to quote Pastor Ward, "Imagine what people could do in life if they did not believe that they were victims." Everything we know is something we learned. Imagine if instead of learning to be victims, we learned to be resilient. Confident. Responsible for our own actions and outcomes.

Victim Culture Leads to Terrible Policy

There's another problem with victim culture: it causes people to advocate for terrible policy solutions to "fix" or "heal" their victimization.

To me, that's why Critical Race Theory (CRT) has become such a hot-button issue. According to the NAACP Legal Defense Fund, CRT is "an academic and legal framework that denotes that systemic racism is part of American society—from education and housing to employment and health care. Critical race theory recognizes that racism is more than the result of individual bias and prejudice. It is embedded in laws, policies, and institutions. . . ."[3]

While a lot of the debate around CRT misstates what CRT actually is, what's undeniable is that, by design, it creates a worldview where everyone has to put on permanent racial lenses to look at every action, every statistic, every student, every employee, and every outcome in every discipline. CRT may take pains to say that individuals aren't racist, but—especially in schools—it sure is getting reported as making white students feel that they are being told they are, and Black students more than occasionally feel like they are being forced into a *victim* role that they don't want. Is it possible that whatever curriculum is being taught, whether CRT or not, has the unintended consequence of creating tension between Black and white students who have grown up in a much more diverse and multicultural world than we did? Is it possible that the children are a lot more accepting and color-blind than we realize, and that the tension and culture of victimization are being manufactured by adults with an adult agenda?

A culture of victimization led to the creation of the San Francisco African American Reparations Advisory Committee, formed to develop a plan to undo "the institutional, City sanctioned harm that has been inflicted upon African American communities." They proposed that anyone who has been incarcerated by "the failed war on drugs" or is the descendant of someone who was, or is a descendant of someone who was enslaved, or experienced lending or housing discrimination, should be eligible for a lump sum payment of $5 million. You read that right, $5 million. Five million is more than the median lifetime earnings for men in America (which is estimated to be $1.8 million for high school graduates and $3.3 million for a college graduate). On top of that, they recommend that the city should make sure that anyone who makes less than $97,000 a year gets a supplemental payment to bring them up to $97,000 a year (which is the city's median income), and that those payments should continue for 250 years—250 years—to address the racial wealth gap in San Francisco.[4]

By the way, I don't even plan on making lump-sum payments to my own children. Both of my sons are hardworking and responsible with money, but when I was putting together my will, I decided that it's just dangerous to give someone a lump sum—regardless of how responsible they are or what capacity they have to handle it. So, I planned several payments over time. After all, anybody can get swindled, make a bad investment, and squander money once. But if someone gets a lump sum, they've only got one chance to get it right.

Let's just say this proposal became law. What would happen? Well, we actually have a pretty decent idea, because there's an experiment that gets conducted once a year that shows exactly what would happen. It's called the NFL Draft. Every year, 262 athletes become millionaires, at least on paper. It's the American Dream for those players: after years of training and hard work, they're now some of the best-paid, most famous people in our society. But many of them are handed that money without the maturity or financial literacy tools needed to manage it. They adopt a media-perpetuated, unrealistic lifestyle that is ultimately unsustainable.

According to *Sports Illustrated*, nearly 80 percent of NFL players file for bankruptcy or experience financial hardship only two years after retiring, at the average age of twenty-seven. I recognize these players aren't getting a handout, they're getting rewarded for a very specific set of skills and talents. My point is that they are receiving something that they're not fully prepared for, and even with all of the supports in place for them, the outcomes aren't good.

Handing out money may assuage somebody's guilt, but it doesn't solve any problems—and may actually create a whole lot more of them. I have said for decades: you do not solve money problems with money. I can't say I'm surprised, but there are already members of the community who would be recipients of those payments who are publicly complaining it is not enough and would just be a "down payment" on what they are owed.

> **Handing out money may assuage somebody's guilt, but it doesn't solve any problems—and may actually create a whole lot more of them. I have said for decades: you do not solve money problems with money.**

And let me be clear, this isn't just about reparations. It's about any direct payment for indirect harm. Look at the many COVID relief programs that were put in place. When the pandemic hit, Democrats and Republicans decided together that our country would pay people not to work, handing out several thousand dollars in "economic impact payments" plus expanded and extended unemployment benefits for people who were out of work. What could go wrong? For starters, people realized they could make more money by not working than they could by working. So, when the world started to open back up again, businesses couldn't find enough workers. This led to all sorts of supply chain disruptions, and it added to inflation.

The bottom line is that if you start guaranteeing equality of outcome regardless of input, you're going to run into big problems. Much more on this coming up.

Victim Culture Leads to a Revenge Cycle

My good friend Dr. James Kimmel is a lecturer in psychiatry at the Yale School of Medicine and the founder and cocreator of the Yale Collaborative for Motive Control Studies.

Dr. Kimmel had a defining moment in his life when he was in high school. He grew up on a farm in central Pennsylvania. He was being bullied, and some of the bullies snuck onto his property and—this sickens me to even think about—shot and killed his beagle.[5] Weeks after that, in the middle of the night, the bullies blew up his mailbox. This time Kimmel rushed out of his house with a gun. In his car he chased the bullies down and cornered them. And in that moment, he could have killed them. I could have mounted a passionate defense on his behalf if he had. (Heck, I'm an animal lover, I've had three wonderful, loving beagles at different times in my life, and there's nothing I'm less tolerant of in this world than bullies.)

Luckily, James's considerable intellect took over and he stopped short. And that's when he decided to become a lawyer and get the right kind of justice. After a very successful career in the law, he started working at the intersection of the law and psychology, and this is where he developed his extremely well-researched and -supported "behavioral addiction" model of violence. He started to see that revenge activates the same neural pathways to the pleasure centers of the brain that opioids, gambling, and video games do. Carrying out an act of revenge, once you have convinced yourself that you have been victimized, creates a "high" much like you would experience if you got a "fix" from a drug. Further, in addition to creating a "high," it acts not just like a drug, but like an *addictive* drug—you want and need more. So, when you see yourself as a victim, you get hooked on looking for revenge. Dr. Kimmel's insight here is profound.

Think about the big picture: we are talking about a brain/behavior/cultural intersection that I believe research will prove to be a major driver in the increased violence we see in our society today.

I have said the extreme ideologues are creating a mindset of "oppressor" and "oppressed." This allows people to distort things in such a way that instead of owning a problem, they become victims.

Consider a situation where someone at their job steals some petty cash from the register. A security guard sees it on the cameras and reports it. The thief gets disciplined or fired, and instead of owning the fact that they made a bad decision, they blame the security guard for getting them fired and seek revenge. A victim culture becomes a revenge culture. And that kind of thinking where individuals never take responsibility for their own actions can, as much as anything, explain the situation our country is in now.

Today more and more people are taught, "Hey, it's not *your* fault! You are a victim here. The system failed you. If they had paid you enough you wouldn't have had to steal that petty cash. It's not your fault! It's their fault. If they cared about you, they would make sure you didn't need to steal. You should get even. You were entitled to that money."

If that sounds ridiculous to you, if you think nobody's logic is that screwed up, I'm sorry to tell you that that example is not some bizarre exaggeration I've made up to prove a point. I can't even begin to tell you how many versions of that victim story I've heard in the last several years. And the more people who believe they are victims, as Dr. Kimmel's research supports, the more they want revenge, and we get stuck in a very destructive cycle.

We see this play out in all sorts of ways. I'll share another example that's not nearly life-and-death but illustrates how this destructive cycle pervades our society: the issue of "cultural appropriation." This is where one culture, the "dominant" culture, takes aspects of another culture, *at the expense of the original culture*. So when Kim Kardashian wears cornrow-style braids, there are those, who are in my opinion looking for more and more ways to play the victim, who accuse her of stealing—of cultural appropriation. Now, she didn't take the hair off of their heads, she just chose a hairstyle, and yes, I know it's a style with cultural significance. What I don't know is: Who is injured by it? You could, on the other hand, embrace the old saying that "imitation is the sincerest form of flattery," which means people tend to copy someone or something they admire. But of course that attitude makes it harder to play the victim.

When somebody popularizes something from another culture, it brings knowledge, honor, and greater understanding and acceptance. Only a victim culture poses that genuine cultural exchange as a victimization of someone that demands revenge. That's the cycle we're in, and it's one we have to get out of.

Stop Witnessing Your Life and Start Living It

When you're a victim, you're also a passenger. Things happen to you. Life happens to you.

Some of you may remember when basketball phenom LeBron James made it to the NBA. At the time, Nike ran a huge advertising campaign with images of LeBron doing the types of things on the basketball court that only LeBron James could do, under the slogan "We Are All Witnesses."

On one level, that slogan was about LeBron's greatness—what a privilege to be able to see one of the greatest of all time.

But on another level, that slogan was a message to the competition—you could watch what LeBron was doing, but you couldn't stop it. You had no control.

But I never thought that was fully true.

A spectator has no control. They're simply observing.

But a witness does have something to offer—their testimony. Their experiences. In fact, in a courtroom, a witness is the *most* powerful person.

Earlier I mentioned that I started a company called Courtroom Sciences to help our clients prepare in courtroom-like conditions for everything they might experience at trial, and understand what juries were thinking, how they were likely to problem-solve for a particular set of facts, and how to determine what mattered to them and what did not.

Based on results, we were very good at what we did. We dealt with every aspect of an upcoming trial. That included case analysis, strategic planning, witness preparation, mock trials, mirror juries who observed the trial and were debriefed nightly, and designing and creating all of the graphics and exhibits needed at trial. We then assisted in jury selection and analyzed the jury's reactions and behaviors during the actual trial, debriefing them post-verdict. At one point, I think we went 487 days without ever closing our graphics department. Through Christmas, Thanksgiving, twenty-four hours a day—there was a constant demand for what we were doing.

There were times we had Learjets on standby to fly the graphics we had created to different trial venues across the country. We changed the game. The same way Tiger Woods made every other golfer realize they had to hit the weight room, we made everyone realize that they had to step up. In our "mock trial" we had a full-blown replica of a very formal federal courtroom where we tested the whole case ahead of time, with people we had paid to be "jurors." Sometimes we would mock-try a case seven or eight times, in front of multiple juries each time. As a result, by the time we got to trial we might have analyzed fifteen to twenty juries deliberating the facts of the case. They taught us what was important and what we had to establish, what we had to prove to win. We learned the other side's case better than they knew it. Eventually we could predict the outcome with a great degree of accuracy, and we were rarely surprised at trial.

Perhaps one of our biggest innovations was something we called the Witness Bill of Rights. The whole idea is that everything in a courtroom is designed to make a witness feel *powerless*. They are in an unfamiliar situation where everyone else seems very comfortable and vested with authority. They're confined to a box. The judge sits up higher than them, surrounded by an impressive state or federal seal. The bailiff wears a uniform and carries a gun. The lawyers know the court reporter by name and get to walk around.

We provided our witnesses with a clear description of their rights. We taught them how to protect and assert themselves without coming off as cocky smartasses. We taught them that *they* in fact were in control and trained them to tell the truth effectively and with power. This was all steeped heavily in psychological dynamics and the psychosocial functioning of the jury's collective personality and the court system as a whole.

I'm telling you this because I think part of why I've been successful in moving from trial sciences into the public sphere is that in many ways, a courtroom is a microcosm of life. The witness's goal in a courtroom is similar to your goal in the world: to present yourself as authentically and powerfully as you can. To deal with situations that might seem stacked against you, where it doesn't seem like you're in control.

We taught our witnesses how to never not be in control. We joked that with enough time and preparation, we could turn Barney Fife into John Wayne. And we did, with several simple tools, techniques, and, yes, rights.

So, to make sure you get your money's worth from this book,

I'm now going to share with you excerpts—and just a few of the insights—from that Witness Bill of Rights. And I'm doing it because the lessons it contains extend far beyond the courtroom.

I think you will find these skills, these "attitudes of approach," relevant in your own life. I've modified them slightly because you're not in a courtroom, you're in the world. But, just like a witness, you may not think you have nearly as much power as you actually have.

You have the right not to know the answer to questions. Saying "I do not know" is not a sign of weakness. Taking time to inform yourself is a sign of strength and agency. In a courtroom, my favorite way for witnesses to express the fact that they don't know something is "I am sorry, I cannot help you there," thereby educating the person who wants something from you that you are indeed trying to be helpful, but you simply cannot help on that particular point. And once stated, never backtrack, never start trying to guess what the answers might be. You either know or you don't.

You have the right not to accept faulty assumptions that are built into the questions you are asked. In court, lawyers have developed several techniques to try to bend you toward their worldview. One principal way they do so is by building assumptions they treat as "factual" information into their position. Much of this "factual information" is either faulty, as in completely untrue, or simply not supported by the facts. In a courtroom, the witness, intent on answering a question, will often unintentionally validate faulty assumptions by simply answering the question that was asked, implicitly accepting the assumption when they should call it out. You have the right and the duty to refuse to accept faulty assumptions. When someone presses you on something, you can "reject the premise" or question the faulty assumption. All you have to say is something like "Before I answer your question I need to be clear that something you rolled into the lead-up is absolutely untrue. With the understanding that it is false,

I can respond to the other part if you would like." You'd be amazed how freeing it is to not be forced to have a discussion on someone else's terms.

➤ Just as a witness has the absolute power to control the demeanor of a deposition, you also have the power to control the demeanor of your interactions. In life, as in a courtroom, you'll come across people who are rude, strident, or accusatory. It takes two to engage in that kind of conduct. In a courtroom, as in life, when you refuse to respond to rude or bullying behavior in kind, it exposes that behavior, and if the person behaving that way has a shred of emotional intelligence, they'll stop. The contrast of your civility in response to someone getting all "red-faced" can be very powerful.

➤ You have the absolute right and power to explain. In a courtroom lawyers try to restrict a witness's answer to "yes" or "no." Nowhere in life do you need to abide by that restriction. You have the right to explain yourself. Now, psychologists agree that the most persuasive way to explain is to respond first and then elaborate, rather than the other way around. It is a far different thing to answer a question, "Yes, with the following explanation . . ." than to answer the question, "My explanation is X," followed by a "yes." The latter answer is interpreted by listeners as evasive, or worse. The former is persuasive and credible—in a courtroom and in life. Answer, *then* explain.

➤ In a courtroom, witnesses have the power and right to see documents they are being asked about and, therefore, have the corresponding duty to ask for them. The same is true in life. If you are being presented with information, or data, or evidence that you're not familiar with, you have the right to ask for it. When you ask for "the receipts," the response you get—whether it's cooperative or evasive—tells you everything! Give yourself permission to take whatever time you need to review the *entire* set of documents or key information you're being presented with, whether that takes thirty seconds or thirty minutes.

You may not ever have to take *the stand*, but I hope these rights help you when it comes time for you take *a stand*.

POLL RESPONSE

Excluding being the victim of an actual crime, how many times in your life have you felt that someone's words and actions made you to feel like your rights or feelings or humanity were activley attacked.

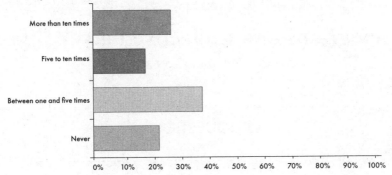

If you answered affirmatively to the preceding question, how long did it take you to move past that initial feeling of injustice?

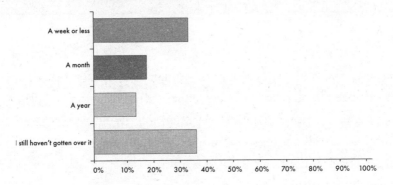

CHAPTER 13

Sociograms and Collective Personality

POLL QUESTION

How often do you engage in debates (online or in real life)
about things you disagree with?
- ☐ Daily
- ☐ Weekly
- ☐ Rarely
- ☐ Never

Many experts who study psychology and human behavior agree that the number one need in all people is acceptance, a sense of belonging. The good news is that if people will just pay attention, we all do belong to something. We are all part of something bigger than ourselves.

Yes, we are all individuals, but each of us is also part of a "collective personality" as well.

Maybe it's at your job where you're part of the staff, maybe it's through your church where you're part of the congregation, or it could even be an online gaming group. Any of the places where you share a common interest or activity with some number of other people. That group will have a collective personality.

Maybe you're part of a very serious group that is dedicated to exonerating innocent prisoners who are on death row, or maybe you're part of an improv comedy group that meets every Tuesday night to develop your comedy writing or stand-up skills.

These groups will have very different collective personalities, but there will be traits and characteristics that define each of them.

Take a moment and list all of the various groups that you are a part of, that you are involved in—centrally or peripherally. Write them down. Now look at your list. My guess is that you'll be surprised at how many different collective personalities you're a part of.

How much you contribute to the group's collective definition is up to you, but what is consistent across them is that every group, every collective of people bound together by any common thread, has that collective personality that defines it. It can be a personality that exists and evolves over the long term, or it can be temporary like a jury in a civil or criminal trial.

I just described Courtroom Sciences Inc., which is the company I cofounded in late 1989 that helped trial lawyers prepare to present their cases to juries in the most effective way possible.

One of the things we focused on right away once we got to trial, usually after months or years of intensive pretrial research, was that juries always developed a very specific collective personality. We knew that if there were twelve people on the jury, there were at least thirteen personalities in that jury box—and probably several more. There were at least twelve individual personalities and one collective personality. Usually there were additional subgroups that had to be figured out and defined.

If we wanted to persuade that jury, we had to figure out all of those dynamics. To do that, we created sociograms. A sociogram is a graphical representation, a chart showing all of the interpersonal relationships a given juror has with other people on the jury. By creating the visual representation, you're able to see who is likely to influence whom and where the power and decision-making is likely to emanate from.

These would often be very complex, and could change over time, but the sociogram would be very instructive when it came to where the lawyers needed to focus their attention and whom the witnesses needed to make eye contact with in order to make sure they got their message across. We saw these sociograms as tools that helped us ensure we weren't just telling the truth, but that we were telling the truth effectively and focusing on the right people. Not all jurors have equal influence when it comes to deliberations, just as not all people in your groups have equal influence.

The decision makers, the biggest influencers, weren't always who you might assume they would be. For example, you might think the jury foreman would be the group's leader. But oftentimes that individual was nothing more than a clerk. The foreman did the paperwork, called for the bailiff if need be, made sure lunch was ordered—but did not necessarily have any influence on decision-making. Only through careful analysis was it possible to find out who was actually in control of or influencing the jury's decision-making process. There's a difference between headship and leadership.

Headship is assigned; leadership is earned. The foreman is usually a headship position, whereas (notice how I slipped a legal-sounding term in there! Ha!) the "leadership" of the jury is whom people gravitate toward because, for any number of reasons, they are respected and trusted by their peers.

Oftentimes in trial, we would recognize that we were really trying our case to a "panel of one." Why? Because some juries had a very charismatic person on the panel to whom others would happily defer. That person, not the lawyer, was the most likely to make the "real" closing argument, and it would happen in the jury room, not the courtroom. Once we recognized that, we made sure that our lawyer focused on that individual and gave him or her the necessary talking points to effectively make that closing argument once they got behind closed doors.

I'm not saying that's how it should be. I'm just telling you that's how it often was.

I'm telling you all of this not because I want you to have a great insight into how a trial really works, but because when I said I believe trials are a microcosm of life, of society, I mean things are very likely to work in a similar fashion within the collective personality groups you or your children find themselves a part of in your real life. What's true in how a jury works in terms of interpersonal dynamics is often true in larger groups throughout our society.

After years and years of working in the litigation arena with so many mock and actual jurors, I came to learn that jury trials are amazing social laboratories. Each member has their own individual personality and consciousness, but they must work together collectively.

Given this understanding of the collective personalities that are created by our various affiliations, can you even begin to imagine how many "collectives" you are part of?

If you want to be influential, for example with your school board regarding what is being taught, how, and when—everything I'm telling you above is *critically relevant* to you having the most impact on those decisions.

Figure out *who is really in charge.* Figure out *who supports whom.* Figure out *what their real motivations are.* Figure out *which facts matter to them and which don't.*

Your school board is just one example, but may not even apply to you. That's why I just asked you to list the places that come to mind where you are part of a group, large or small, and what part you play in defining the personality of the group.

Now think about how many of those groups you're a part of that have a leader, spokesperson, or outspoken activist who at least publicly defines the collective personality of that group. Ask yourself if the positions they take are truly congruent with how you think, feel, and believe.

Does this person or persons really represent you?

Did they consult you?

At one time were the positions taken more consistent with your beliefs than they are now—perhaps the group has evolved and things feel as if they've gotten "out of hand"?

Is this a person or a person who got caught up in the publicity of the cause?

Are they someone who never saw a camera or microphone they didn't like? Have they perhaps forgotten the rule that "too much time in the spotlight fades the suit"?

I wrote earlier about law students at Stanford who shouted down a judge who was there as an invited speaker. This brought significant negative attention to *all* Stanford Law students, and even resulted in a handful of judges saying they would ban Stanford Law graduates from their clerkships. Many of the students interviewed after the fact stated that they felt cheated and misrepresented by activist classmates who did not speak for them.

They blamed the extreme students on both ends of the spectrum who did not represent the 80 or 90 percent of the students between the two extremes.

However, the students between the extremes are guilty of that passivity that can be construed as implicit endorsement, as explained earlier. They did not make their feelings known, so by default it was assumed, perhaps unfairly, that those who were yelling the loudest spoke for them.

How about you?

Are you even loosely tied to any groups or organizations that are taking radical positions in a way that could paint you with that brush?

Because if you fail to speak up, you could be.

"We" can no longer allow the Tyranny of the Fringe to be, by default, the only message heard.

This may be true with your job, your church, your children's school or school board, or anywhere that a self-chosen few speak for the many.

Whatever the collection of people, some*thing* or some*one* will act to create an *energy*, an attitude, an identity that helps define that group.

Sometimes a certain *vibe* will exist, and someone or some new faction might come in and really change the chemistry in a good or bad way. Take a minute to think about some groups you may be part of that have that well-defined "collective personality."

Has the group you're thinking about been a good thing in your life, or has it been a burden, an emotional prison? Stepping back and viewing things that way, you may or may not want to remain a part of every collective personality of which you are a member.

You are also an element—albeit a smaller one—of the collective personality of many larger groups. Maybe you are Texan, Floridian, Virginian, Catholic, or vegan. Even, yes (for most of you, I'm guessing), an American? Think about the American *vibe*. Has it changed significantly in the last few years? As a member of the "collective," did you push it? Were you even aware that a shift in value or ideology was happening? Were you "pulled along"? Were you afraid to speak out? Can you take pride in owning your role?

Whatever the collection of people, some*thing* or some*one* will act to create an *energy*, an attitude, an identity that helps define that group.

You may think, "No way am I connected to someone who lives two or three thousand miles away! How would that even work?" Well, you are and it does work. You see it in the stock market every day. There's an old saying that markets run on confidence. The collective mood in America changes and people buy or sell stock and drive the market up or down.

You see it in the polls concerning political performance. You don't know how someone three thousand miles away is answering a poll question, but you "feel" the shift in optimism or pessimism.

President George W. Bush had the highest rating of any president, ever, right after the attacks that took place on September 11, 2001. There were no Democrats or Republicans, only Americans—and nearly everyone supported our president. By the end of his presidency, he registered one of the lowest.

President Biden as of this writing is approaching historic lows, as did President Trump before him. It's not like people are having secret meetings to discuss how "the collective" feels, but in ways large and small, through individual conversations and broadcast messages, there is lots of shared input.

We also see the collective personality of entire generations changing. Compared to that of the Baby Boomers, the personality of the current generation is markedly different. The current generation is dating later, feels much less urgency to get their driver's license, is having sex later, marrying later, and moving out on their own later. I'm not saying any of that is good or bad; I'm just pointing out that it is collectively different.

What is true of generations is also true of geographies. Take the city of Portland, Oregon. A lot of people settle in Portland because they feel it reflects their values. Creative. Tolerant. A little quirky. But merge those individual personalities into a collective personality and I'm guessing the people of Portland didn't sign up for a collective personality where ten thousand cars a year get stolen and the police do next to nothing.[1] Though they are individually compassionate to those less well-off, they didn't sign up for a collective situation in which the city has been overrun by homelessness. In fact, we know they didn't, because when they saw it, they got rid of the leaders they had elected.

All these individual personalities went to Portland for a reason. But then someone, or a few people, defined the narrative and values of that collective group. Someone defined the collective personality that may not have reflected the individual personalities.

Something similar is happening in America. We've created a collective personality that the majority of us aren't comfortable with. Collectively, we're simply not solving problems. Look at crime, for example. There's a joke about two people who come across someone who has been mugged, lying in a ditch, bloodied and battered. The first person says, "We need to find who did this." And the second says, "Yes, *that person* needs help." The joke is that the passerby is trying to solve a deeper problem without addressing the immediate problem.

If I back the car out of the driveway and run over your foot, your foot doesn't care whether I did it on purpose or if it was an accident, whether I was kicked as a child and have been trying to get revenge on feet ever since. You still have a smashed foot. And if there's some way for me to suppress foot-running-over behavior, that needs to happen. At some point, you can figure out why someone's running over toes. But at the same time, you've got to stop them from running over toes.

This isn't some silly example. In our country, we've seen a resurgence of muggings and random violent aggressions. And clearly, the people perpetrating these acts are not well and they're not the mainstream. But how we respond to that sort of thing as a society says a lot.

A portion of our society has been described as woke because they're saying that the people who are doing this—they're victims themselves. They've been damaged. They've been hurt. And we can't deal with them as criminals because of it.

Well, to me, it's like trying to fix a psychological problem medically or a medical problem psychologically. You have to deal with psychological problems psychologically and medical problems medically. And sometimes they intertwine. But look, there are a lot of people doing a lot of dysfunctional things in our society right now because they've had a dysfunctional life. No question about that. But we have principles in this society, and there have to be consequences for violating them.

We have to look at our roles in rebuilding the society in which we want to live. And that starts with the most important building block—family.

POLL RESPONSE

How often do you engage in debates (online or in real life) about things you disagree with?

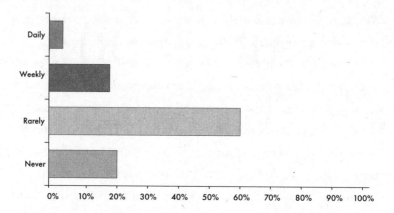

I am disheartened to see the number of people who said they never or rarely engage in debates. I asked this question here because sometimes it can be harder to raise concerns or disagreements in groups or organizations that you're a member of or with people you often do agree with. But that's what shaping or redirecting a collective personality you see going astray requires. It requires you to raise your hand and say, "I don't like where this is going." And before we finish this book, I hope I give you the confidence and empirical data to feel comfortable doing that.

PART THREE

Family, Faith, and Community

About twenty years ago, I wrote a book called *Family First*. In it, I wrote that "people enter our family's world from all walks of life, teachers, coaches, extended family, school bullies, the all-powerful peers and others. Some are well-intentioned and some not. These people may have priorities and values that are different from our own, and they can tremendously affect how our children think, feel, and behave now, as well as who they become as adults. Bombardment from a massive and slick media can undermine morals and values in even the strongest of families if purposeful care is not taken to control and counteract those messages."

Boy, when I wrote that I had no idea what was headed our way.

The other thing I wrote was that socialization is one of the most important jobs a family has. When the family fails to provide the healthy nurturing that children need, the impact on their lives can be destabilizing and cheat them out of the chance to be the best person they can be. Children who are not socialized have problems in the world. They do not respect the authority, hierarchy, or boundaries of their parents. They have poor impulse control. They can be selfish and extremely demanding.

Our current generation of children have undergone an unprecedented sabotage of their socialization, self-worth, self-esteem, and educational attainment.

This assault on their well-being occurred when our government shut down the schools during the pandemic, knowing full well that they were at minimal risk and already suffering the highest levels of depression, anxiety, and loneliness since those measures have been recorded.

I am not naïve. I understand that there is such a thing as "unintended consequences." I'm not such a conspiracy theorist as to suggest that anyone was "out to get" our children. I am also cognizant of the concept of "gross negligence." Legal experts will tell you when someone behaves in such a reckless way as to rise to the level of a wanton disregard for the outcome of their actions, the law deems that conduct to be tantamount to intentionality. In other words, they behave so recklessly that it is considered in the eyes of the law as the same as if they did it intentionally, on purpose.

I have a hard time not defining those circumstances just that way, and I suspect many of you do too. I said so publicly at the time, more than once. April 2020. May 2020. December 2020. I wasn't shy about it.

And people weren't shy about coming after me at the time as if I were insane or a heretic. It's interesting to note that not one single person or outlet bothered to come back and apologize or retract their slanderous comments once it was clear that everything I said was 100 percent true. (It's okay, I wasn't holding my breath.)

I go into greater depth on all this in our chapter on rationality of thought. My point in bringing it up here is that your child, whether they were in kindergarten, college, or anywhere in between, has been impacted. There has never been a more important time for families to close ranks and rally around these young people to help them close the gap and regain what has been lost mentally, emotionally, and academically.

The only way that can be achieved is by your family becoming "purposeful."

If you and your family are doing exactly what you were doing before this government-imposed quarantine, if you have not consciously chosen to sit down, make, and activate an observable plan to deal with the gaps that have been created, then you are missing the boat.

By "observable" I mean, if the people who know your family best can't observe your patterns and readily see that priorities and behaviors have changed, you are very likely falling short of what is necessary.

Overcoming the gaps in functioning is going to require everyone in the family unit working together.

The things you might have to do include replacing the habit of spending too much time on social media or the internet in general, setting aside scheduled times to discuss emotionality, seeking professional help in the form of therapy or tutoring or study groups, programming your young people's lives to reengage socially and competitively, consciously reinvigorating your faith-based life, and on and on and on.

Every situation is different and driven by the needs of the young people in your family. Parents, I recognize that you have needs as well and you can't give away what you don't have. This puts pressure on you to make sure you're getting what you need, because the reality is that as parents, there are certain things you can delegate but there is nothing you can abdicate.

> **As I have said, it is my belief that the family unit is the building block of our country, and the family unit in America is under attack.**

As I have said, it is my belief that the family unit is the building block of our country, and the family unit in America is under attack. And I am far from alone. It was Pope John Paul II who said, "As the family goes, so goes the nation and goes the whole world in which we live."

That does not mean that something or someone or some organization is sitting in the bushes taking potshots at you and your loved ones. What it means is that conditions and circumstances are evolving in such a way that your family unit is getting pushed off center stage and down the priority ladder.

The family is just like a garden. If you go out into a field and clear a place for a garden, you till the ground and clear away all of the weeds and rocks, you plant seeds and water them and fertilize them until they begin to grow, and you continue to weed, and water, and tend to those plants, and then you have a garden.

If you cease to attend to it, if you don't go out on a regular basis and continue to water and fertilize the plants and fight off the weeds, the garden will soon get swallowed up. You won't even be able to see where it once existed. It has to be nurtured, tended to, and protected. Your family is the same way. And it went through some very harsh times. Call the pandemic a drought, call social media a flood—the point is that your garden needs serious nurturing and tending to. It will not heal itself on its own.

I had—and have—more to say about all of this. But reading now what I wrote back in *Family First*, I want to offer an addendum, an update.

When I was writing that, I was concerned that the dysfunction of unsocialized children can contaminate the family. Today I would argue that the decline of the family can contaminate *society*.

Indeed, the very building blocks of our society—family, faith, and community—are crumbling. And we need to strengthen them, because they're the foundation on which everything else is built.

CHAPTER 14

The Family Is Under Attack

POLL QUESTIONS

To what extent do you think the strength and closeness of the family unit actually impact the strength and unity of the country as a whole?

- ☐ Very
- ☐ Somewhat
- ☐ Not very
- ☐ Not at all

To what extent do you think the strength and closeness of the family unit in America have declined from the last generation to the current generation?

- ☐ Very
- ☐ Somewhat
- ☐ Not very
- ☐ Not at all

Picture a massive category 5 tornado spinning across the landscape. You can see it, a dark funnel cloud, twisting, accelerating. It grinds up anything and everything in its path. Every so often there is a flash of light or an explosion as it uproots a power line, or picks up a truck, spins it around and flings it out, causing even more damage. If you have never experienced a tornado, you are fortunate. I know you have seen the aftermath on the news, with homes wrecked and lives left in shambles. Trust me when I tell you that in person, it's even worse.

That's how I picture what's happening to the American family today. We are in a vicious cycle that is spinning families out of control.

Here's the spinning tornado for families: The decline of religion's influence on society has led to divorce and cohabitation becoming more acceptable. Divorce and cohabitation becoming more acceptable leads to fewer, later marriages. Fewer, later marriages mean fewer children. Fewer children leads to less organized religion membership and attendance, and less organized religion combined with more children of divorce means fewer marriages—and around and around we go. It's all linked.

And here's the debris that's getting thrown off: more children of single parents and broken homes, who then have much worse education, life, and health outcomes, which imposes a cost on all of us.[1] By the way, it's worse for the single parents too. As one example, single parents are 1.3 times more likely to have a heart condition than partnered parents.[2]

Fewer children overall slows the economy, which means less opportunity for everyone.[3]

When the traditional family breaks down, everything starts breaking down.

> **When the traditional family breaks down, everything starts breaking down.**

Let's look a little deeper at what's happening, starting with some stunning numbers on marriage and family in America.

In 1960, at the height of the baby boom after World War II, 5 percent of children were born to unwed parents. By 1980, that number had more than tripled, reaching 18 percent.

In 2016, a whopping 40 percent of children in the United States were born to women who were single moms or living with a nonmarital partner.[4]

In the 1960s, 73 percent of all children were living in a family with two married parents who were in their first marriage. By 1980, 61 percent of children were living in this type of family.

Percent of Children Living with Two Parents in First Marriage

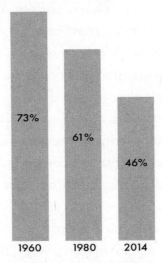

Percent of Children Born to Unwed Parents

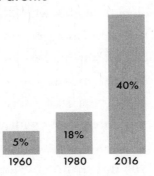

Today, 46 percent of children—less than half!—are living in a family with two married parents in their first marriage.[5]

So kids today are a lot more likely to be born to an unwed mother and a lot less likely to live in a family with two married parents on their first marriage.

The share of children living in a two-parent household is at the lowest point in more than half a century. In fact, more than four in ten Black children live only with their mother. In fact, this is the *most common* living arrangement for Black children. Compare that to two out of every ten Hispanic children, one out of every ten white children, and one out of every fourteen Asian children.[6]

The United States has the world's highest rate of children living in single-parent households. And for a lot of reasons, that is *not* a statistic where we want to be leading the world.

Here's another statistic that is actually scary in two ways: estimates suggest that about 39 percent of children will have had a mother in a cohabiting relationship by the time they turn twelve; and by the time they turn sixteen, almost half will have experience with their mother cohabiting.[7]

At first glance, you would think that sounds good—a stable household with a mother and a father.

But cohabitation and marriage are very different things.

And cohabitation with a nonbiological relative puts a child at much higher risk for abuse than any other form of living situation.

A child with a biological mother who is living with a man who is not the child's father is 33 times more likely to suffer abuse.[8] And fatal assaults of young children by stepfathers are over 100 times greater than those by genetic fathers.[9] In fact, abuse or even murder by a step-parent is so common that it even has a name: "the Cinderella effect."[10]

So, to sum it up: children living with their married biological parents have the lowest rate of abuse and neglect, whereas those living with a single parent who had a partner living in the household have the highest rate.[11]

Meanwhile, in America, we've reached what some would call an interesting tipping point, and I would call it a dangerous one. It's now more common to have cohabited than to have married. Meaning, more

adults between the ages of 18 and 44 have lived with a romantic partner than have ever been married. You might say, "Well, a lot of people
living with someone are *basically* married—isn't that the same thing?"

No, no it's not.

Yes, it's true that most people who have cohabited with someone
have only ever—and will only ever—live with that one partner. But a
significant share, 14 percent, will have three or more partners. Cohabiting isn't marriage, because you can just walk out the door. Unlike a
marriage, there's no legal or societal obligation to work through differences. Nobody made a vow to stand together for richer or poorer,
in sickness and in health.

Why so many cohabitators? Because they're the children of divorce
themselves.

Adult children of divorce are 47 percent more likely to be cohabit-
ers, compared with those who were raised in intact, married families.[12]

Divorce has played a key role in reducing marriage and increasing
cohabitation—*a generation later.*

And there's a lot of divorce. You've probably heard the statistic
that 50 percent of marriages end in divorce. That statistic is actually
a little misleading, because it includes a lot of those short, first-time
"starter" marriages, as well as the folks who are serial divorcers. I have
two sisters who were married eleven times between them. They've
probably skewed the statistics a bit! In reality, it's more like 25 percent
of first marriages end in divorce, and nearly three-quarters of second
marriages end in divorce.[13] Still, that's a lot, and this is a concern,
because the children of divorce have a higher risk of developing a vari-
ety of mental health conditions, an unhealthy weight and BMI gain,
and suffer more anxiety and depression.[14]

Divorce and parental separation also created an increased risk for
child and adolescent adjustment problems, including academic diffi-
culties like lower grades or dropping out of school, disruptive behaviors, and substance abuse problems.

Children of divorced or separated parents are also one and a half to two times more likely to engage in risky sexual behavior, live in poverty, and experience their own family instability.[15]

Yes, there are some marriages—so-called "high-conflict marriages"—in which a partner or a child is at risk of violence, or is under constant psychological stress. People need to get out of those marriages, and the children benefit from it.[16]

But in almost every other case, the divorce is detrimental to the children.

How Do We Stop the Tornado?

We've got to stop this tornado. And standing in front of it waving our arms won't do. But there are some steps we can take. In my books *Relationship Rescue* and *Family First*, I write extensively about what individuals, couples, and families can do.

Here I want to talk about what we as a society can do.

The first, and most important, thing we need to do is stop subsidizing societally destructive behavior.

Second, we need to speak up for marriage. For a long time, marriage was strongly institutionalized. By that, I mean there were clear roles partners were supposed to play, and norms they were supposed to adhere to. Marriage had a very practical aspect to it—it's what enabled you to survive in society. Today marriage is more about love, romance, and personal choice. It's less of a practical necessity, and more of a symbolic meaning.[17]

Another reason sociologists say that there are fewer marriages now is what they call less associational life and rising affluence, and what I call "attempting to buy a spouse."[18] I don't mean like a mail-order bride—the theory here is that there have been declines in family and community, but an increase in wealth, so people are "buying" the things that used to be part of a marriage partnership. Paying a non-relative to cook, or clean, or provide childcare. The idea is that more money has made it less important to have a spouse, a coparent, or in-laws. I don't buy it, but that's the theory.

The reason I don't buy it is that marriage provides something that you can't buy. At any price. Ever.

My wife, Robin, would be pleased to hear me say this, because I'm not terribly expressive emotionally. But I feel strongly that marriage provides something unique and important. It provides you with a partner who is someone you feel safer with than anyone else in the world.

You're proud of them, and it matters to you if they're proud of you.

You care where they are, and it matters to you that they care where you are.

It's someone you can interact with in a way and at a level that you can't with anybody else in your life. Who you share things with that you don't share with anyone else in the world.

It provides the support you need to rise and a soft place if you fall.

Marriage is curative.

It is healing.

People who are happily married have a different biochemistry within their brain and body than people who are alone or in a bad marriage.

Men who are married live longer. (Even though I joke that marriage sometimes makes them more willing to die.)

That's not to say that you should just waltz into marriage like you're skipping through a field of flowers. Marriages take work; relationships take work. I recommend counseling (or a close reading of my book *Relationship Rescue*) ahead of time.

But at the end of the day, all of the reasons people cite for not getting married (the sociologist Ulrich Beck calls them "individualization trends")—prioritizing self-fulfillment, happiness, career—are reasons I think run in favor of marriage!

Third, and this is related: we need to encourage *more men to be men*. We need more men to see that there's a benefit in life to being a responsible provider. In fact, if you're a man, one of the best ways to get a raise and increase your wages *is to get married*.

One of the theories behind the fewer marriages is that fewer men clear the bar to be worth marrying.[19] The irony here is that marriage makes men better men. When men have a wife or children to support, they become more focused on the job market. Studies show that married men typically work harder and more successfully. They are less likely to be fired, and they make about $16,000 more than their single peers with otherwise similar backgrounds.

This is what economists call men's "marriage premium." Studies find that both in the United States and other developed countries, married men earn between 10 and 40 percent more than otherwise comparable single men. A study of identical twins found an earnings increase of about one-quarter for the twin who was married. The data clearly show that the financial return on investment of marriage is substantial for men.[20]

So, if we want to stop the tornado and save families, we have to stop subsidizing the destruction of the family unit, start advocating for marriage, and get more men to step up to the plate and be men.

POLL RESPONSE

To what extent do you think the strength and closeness of the family unit actually impact the strength and unity of the country as a whole?

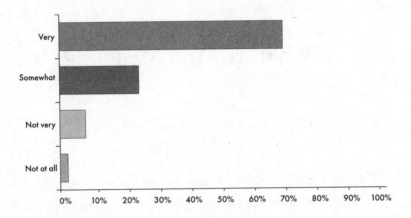

To what extent do you think the strength and closeness of the family unit in America have declined from the last generation to the current generation?

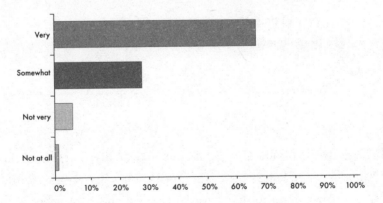

I was so glad to see that so many people acknowledge that the family unit is key to the strength of the country. But almost the same number said the strength of the family unit has declined. That means, at least in my view, it should go on the top of our to do list.

CHAPTER 15

What Are You Modeling?

POLL QUESTION

Is there a generational legacy that you believe impacts your family life today? If so, how often do you consciously work to embrace and enhance it if it is positive or eliminate it if it is negative?

☐ Always

☐ Very often

☐ Sometimes

☐ Never

Throughout this book, I have written repeatedly that the backbone of America is the family unit. This country has been built around the family—think of how many towns were anchored by family farms and family businesses. Across generations and until quite recently, the family unit lived and grew together. The family unit, and the multigenerational family home, were where you were born and raised, and often returned to in your old age. Throughout your life, family provided the "soft place to fall." Demographic and geographic patterns have changed some of that, and dysfunction has certainly undercut it, but for most, the family unit has been the most consistent, most constant institution in people's lives.

I think some of the attacks on family that I have written about are purposeful, coming from those who, out of a desire to redefine the face of America, want to break down the whole concept of a nuclear family. Even the biological underpinnings of motherhood and fatherhood have come under attack recently.

Other trends at odds with the concept of family are such realities as the erosion of religious affiliation, a very family-oriented element of our culture, which has dropped below the 50 percent participation level for the first time ever.

Another trend has been the undeniable immersion, especially by the current generation, into the virtual world where electronic devices and social media platforms, programmed to be addictive, have competed for and crowded out family time, supplanting time and space that previously was dedicated to family members. You know this in your bones, but here are the numbers:

- Although most apps require a child to be 13 years old to use them, one-third of children between the ages of 7 and 9 and half of children between the ages of 10 and 12 are on a social media platform.
- 54 percent of children feel that their parents check their own devices too often, and 32 percent of children feel unimportant when their parents are distracted by their phones.
- 69 percent of parents and 78 percent of teens check their devices hourly.
- 59 percent of parents say that they feel their teens are addicted to their mobile devices, and 50 percent of teens agree![1]

This is one reason why I have repeatedly said to parents, "You will not be the only voice in your child's ear, so you must certainly be the best voice your child's ear."

These electronic addictions result in huge time shifts away from family interactions. Even when family members are together, you see the intrusion of devices. Next time you go to a restaurant and see a family supposedly having dinner "together," pay attention to how many members of the family, including Mom and Dad, are on their devices, not making eye contact or having real conversations. (I must make a parenthetical comment here. I was actually dictating this passage of the book, and we have become so electronic/virtual/computer defined that when I dictated "eye contact" the voice recognition program defaulted to "iContact!" And I repeated it several times, and it continued to give me "iContact." How sad is it that "eye contact" has become so obsolete that it's unrecognizable even to the dictionary inside the dictation program?!)

> **This is one reason why I have repeatedly said to parents, "You will not be the only voice in your child's ear, so you must certainly be the best voice your child's ear."**

This is an especially relevant and salient point in my view because of our earlier discussion about today's coddled generation. Are the voices in your children's ears speaking the truth? Are they espousing the values you believe will bring them the greatest long-term joy and fulfillment in their lives? Or are those voices pumping them full of the ideas of those who see America through a filter that distorts reality and changes a child's perception from one of clarity about how the world really works into a fiction of how others *wish* it worked?

The philosophies being pushed by some of the loudest voices on the internet are so fanciful, so based on an idea of "everything for free" and "everyone bends to your will" wonderland, that a cruel shock will await anyone seduced by such messaging who eventually has to enter the real world.

All of this is to say that when I write about "being who you are on purpose," I hope and pray that who you are and who you wish to be includes committing to an active role in your family, as well as dedicating yourself to serving as a model of good behavior for your family members.

Such basics as family time, family leadership, family unity, and values are worthy priorities. Allowing them to be replaced with brain-numbing time spent on electronic devices and investing in false group affiliations with people you don't really know is a devastating mistake that parents can't afford to make, or to let their children make. This is an insidious and silent seduction with no real basis in shared experiences. These allegiances seduce us with glitz, glamour, and lifestyles that are unattainable because they are manufactured fantasies created with scripts, editing, and a lot of photoshopping.

I promise you when you are in need, physically, financially, emotionally, or in any other real-world fashion, family shows up. Clickbait influencers, bots, and photoshopped people you have never met do not.

If you doubt me, message some of your TikTok or Instagram friends and let them know you need a "chemo buddy" to sit with you for hours each week, or someone to help you move from your third-floor walk-up apartment. See how many of them step up and volunteer for any of those not-so-glamorous requests.

If you are a parent or a grandparent in the role of parent, I have a special message for you. As I said in a previous book, *Family First*, children may roll their eyes and at least pretend they're not listening, but whether they are or not, you can bet they are always watching. So, the question you must ask yourself is: "What exactly are they seeing as they watch me? What example am I setting in the way I live my life?"

It just makes common sense that the most powerful role model in any child's life is the same-sex parent, and that the second-most-powerful role model is the other-sex parent. You are the ones who are there from the beginning, you are there the most, you are the ones who have the ability to write on the slate of who they become.

Clearly there are genetic influences, but when it comes to social learning such as values and beliefs, you're in the best position to have the most powerful influence. And remember, it's never too late. Sometimes you parent and sometimes you "re-parent." The one thing I'm pretty sure of is that you never completely finished the job! Even when they grow up and move on and move out, and even when they start their own families, if you've done a good job and you have open lines of communication, you *still* parent; you might just do it long-distance. If you're like me, you will consider that opportunity a blessing. I know I certainly welcome those calls when they come and you can bet Robin does.

You may say, and if you're part of the vast majority of parents in America you would be correct, "Well, you know, we don't fight in front of the children, and we certainly were not vicious, evil abusers— child protective services would not take our children if they were a fly on the wall and watched our parenting. We probably haven't been perfect, but we always came from a place of love."

That's great, sincerely. I mean, it's what's expected, but it's still great that you aren't or weren't overtly toxic. But you must also consider what you might be modeling that is much more mundane and subtler, but still negative. You also need to consider what you are *not* modeling that you could and should be if you want to set your children up for the biggest chance for success, however they might define that.

If you're modeling apathy, if you're modeling "being a sellout," that would be cheating them terribly. I know words like *sellout* sound really harsh, but if you go to work every day and you come home saying things like "Oh my God, the same old grind. I just hate that job. They don't appreciate me. I hate my life," but you keep doing it nonetheless, you are not modeling agency.

If you are in an abusive relationship mentally, emotionally, or physically or you're in an emotionally barren one, but you do nothing about it, you are modeling for your son or daughter the idea that's what your life ends up being when you make it to adulthood. You are modeling that's what you settle for.

If you model the path, the pattern, the expectation that what you do is go to school, learn, take a job you hate, and grind through it until you die, that may seem like your reality, but it is certainly not inspirational for them. What kind of role model is that for a child: a parent who lives a passionless, uninvolved, gray, drab, sellout life?

Is that the message you want to send? I think you know the answer.

Do you complain about the government but do nothing about it? Do you complain about the quality of your life and policies that impact you but do nothing about it? Do you read about cancel culture, things being taught or not taught in schools, homelessness, gun violence, climate issues, crime and punishment or the lack thereof, and any number of other cultural issues but never do or say anything about them? Do you have friends who you think are way off base on some issue but remain silent or "smile and nod" in front of your children when they know you feel decidedly different?

If so, ask yourself, first, "Am I being authentic with myself?" and then, "What kind of role model am I being for my children?"

This is important because research tells us children are very likely to emulate their parents once they are on their own. Just as an example, it is well documented that mothers who remain in abusive relationships often have daughters who wind up in similar relationships.[2]

If I am causing you to assess what kind of model you are being for your children, that's a good thing. But making changes will not be easy. There are many reasons why it's difficult to make changes. One is that behaviors become habitual. On an even deeper level, everybody, to some degree, is a product of parental or generational legacy.

As I've said, parents are powerful influences on their children and your parents were a powerful influence on you. You have to decide whether you want to be a prisoner of your past, or whether you want to rewrite your family value system and consciously choose to end a negative generational legacy if one exists.

I'm not assuming that you had a negative upbringing. If you were raised by a wonderful, loving, nurturing parent, that's great. You want to carry that forward. Emulate everything you possibly can. But if you did not, if you had a negative upbringing or if it was mixed in some way, you have to choose to be who you are on purpose. Choose what you want to carry forward and choose what you want to leave behind.

Don't saddle your children by perpetuating the generational curse that they have to carry forward and will one day burden *their* children with. Decide it stops now; it stops with you.

This comes full circle. I have said that the backbone of America is the family unit. So, the stronger the family unit, the more the family withstands the attacks they are now under, the more we fortify this country.

You have to clean your own house first. Strengthen your family. Stop the generational curse. Fight off the onslaught of the internet and the electronic intrusion of these cultlike addictive devices and reclaim your family. It's like drawing a line in the sand or, even more symbolically, flying the American flag in your front yard to say, "This family proudly supports America!" That is how important families are to America, and we need that resurgence of passionate support.

To be proactive in leading your family and in supporting America, you can start by writing down five things that you have carried forward from your childhood that you think are positive, and five things you have carried forward that you think are negative. The negative just goes on your to-do list.

I'll give you one example of each from my life. My father was a violent alcoholic. There was chaos and emotional and financial instability in my home, so I would not want to carry any of that forward.

We were often so poor we couldn't pay our utilities or buy groceries, and there were so many unknowns and so much unpredictability.

Which is why I made the decision to never drink. I thought, there's no decision to make about how much is too much, how much is interfering, if you decide just not to do it at all.

On the positive side, and interestingly enough also involving my father, he was the hardest-working person I ever knew. He had no quit in him. I decided to emulate that work ethic. I carried that forward and instilled that into both of my boys. We maintain a balance but we're not afraid of hard work.

Hopefully those examples will help get you started. I can't overstate how important I think it would be to sit down as a family and talk about what we have covered in this chapter. I know it sounds corny and old-fashioned to have a family meeting—but the more awkward it feels, the more necessary it probably is. Your family will benefit and so will your country.

POLL RESPONSE

Is there a generational legacy that you believe impacts your family life today? If so, how often do you consciously work to embrace and enhance it if it is positive or eliminate it if it is negative?

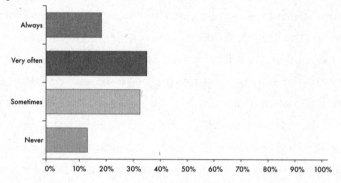

The response to this question is very encouraging because it tells me we're really thinking about this. And I think it does need to be on our minds. We need to be cognizant of what's going on in our families. It's certainly something I've thought a lot about, and I hope you continue to do the same.

CHAPTER 16

The Dangerous Erosion of Faith

POLL QUESTION

How often do you attend an organized religious service?
- ☐ Weekly or more
- ☐ Monthly
- ☐ Once or twice a year
- ☐ Never

At the outset of this book, I said I was going to challenge you to get to know yourself, your beliefs, and your opinions really well so you can be who you are on purpose. And right now, the area I'm asking you to focus on is your faith. Don't worry; I'll go first.

I was raised in the Southern Baptist Church and was baptized in the Village Baptist Church in Oklahoma City when I was thirteen years old. In the Baptist Church, you are baptized the same way John the Baptist baptized Jesus in the Jordan River—by dunking him completely under the water.

I had buddies and teammates who were Methodists. We, of course, compared notes on our experiences. When I described walking into a tank that looked like it belonged in an aquarium and getting the "full dunk," their first response was "NO WAY!" Then the questions flowed: Were you in your suit? Did you get water up your nose? Was it cold? They then shared their tales of their "more sophisticated" baptisms, which involved just pouring some water on them. They pretended to look down on us Baptists. As they used to jokingly say in Oklahoma, Methodists are just Baptists who can read. The ribbing and jokes were all in good fun after a serious rite that, although administered differently, actually served to connect us.

But I *could* read, and read I did. I studied the Bible just as I studied all important things, then and now. Even at a young age I tested what I was reading and was being told. I didn't take things at face value or for granted.

Early on, I talked to the pastor in a pretty unusual way. I'd challenge him, "Do you think I'm stupid because I'm thirteen?"

I've got to give him credit, because he wasn't a fire-and-brimstone kind of guy and didn't blow me off or accuse me of being disrespectful. He'd smile and get ready for what was coming and say, "I don't think you're stupid. I think you're one of the smarter kids in this church."

And so I'd say, "Well, then why do I need to come back here every week? Because you pretty much say the same thing. You rotate scripture and topics, but I pretty much got it after the first year: behave yourself, do a good job, worship the Lord. Gotcha. I could give you the sermon."

He would reply, "Really? Give me one."

So I'd give him an impromptu sermon and he'd ask me if I knew what it all meant, and we'd go back and forth, and when I showed I understood it, I asked my question again: "Why do I have to come back?"

Finally he said, "You know why? Because you need to come in here, away from the rest of the world, to be still and focus on the

Lord, even if it's just an hour a week. You need to hit the reset button. Even if you know everything I'm going to say, which you don't even if you think you do, you and your family need that time to reset in the presence of the Lord, even if it's just for an hour a week. You're better off for it."

I remember sort of begrudgingly agreeing with him. Going to church did give me the opportunity to thank God for the many blessings of life. I have since learned in my study of human psychology how important an attitude of gratitude is to our well-being. Faith and science are certainly in agreement on this point.

Going to church gave me the opportunity to acknowledge my own shortcomings, my sins. Doing that helped me do better, be better, feel better. As you have no doubt heard me say, as Dr. Phil, "you can't change what you don't acknowledge." Going to church, and thus drawing closer to God, gives you both the opportunity and the motivation to acknowledge the things about yourself that you wish to change. There is good in each of us. It is that part of us that helps us resist temptation to do wrong. It is the part of us that causes us to be fair, to be honest, to be dependable and caring.

But there is also evil in each of us too. Every day, there are a million competitions and one of them, good or evil, will win, and one will lose. The winner will be the one we feed the most. I came to see that time spent building a relationship with our Creator is lunchtime for good.

Only later did I start seeing the scientific evidence that backed up that feeling.

The benefit of having faith in God is not some vague notion. It is demonstrably helpful. Our Founders saw that. They knew they wanted a separation of church and state—they didn't want us governed by *any single religion*—but at the same time they felt religion in general was essential if we were going to have good and decent citizens, and that good and decent citizens were essential to a successful country.* That's why you see references to God woven into the fabric and the words of our founding documents. It is as important to us now, in continuing to be a great country, as it was to them then. Consider how many of our key national documents and oaths invoke God. The Declaration of Independence talks about "Nature's God" and our "creator." Take any oath of office and you'll conclude with the words "so help me God." If you've ever seen a case argued before the United States Supreme Court, you'll hear the last words of the clerk in announcing the justices, "God save the United States and this honorable court." Just turn over that dollar bill and read what is written on the back—"In God We Trust."

Perhaps most importantly, read the First Amendment to our Constitution, which granted rights and protections for the worship of God.

But did you know that our commitment to organized religion has been on the decline for some time? Right around 2020, church membership in the United States dropped below 50 percent for the first time in our history.[1]

Even as our population grows, somewhere between six thousand and ten thousand churches close down every year.[2] Many cathedrals in Europe are empty tombs. If people go at all, it's to view them as relics, as museums. But when it comes to actual services, there are more bodies in the crypts than in the pews!

That is a sad state of affairs. And we are not far behind unless we do something about it.

---

* George Washington wrote that the only being to whom Americans owed an explanation of their religious beliefs was God.

Church Membership Among U.S. Adults Now Below 50%

Do you happen to be a member of a church, synagogue, or mosque?
 % Yes, member

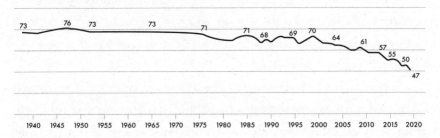

Based on annual aggregated data, usually based on two surveys
GALLUP

    This is not to say that we don't believe in God, or the Almighty, or some higher power—most of us still do.

    But we're leaving behind *organized* religion—which I'm defining as a structured system of faith or worship, especially one followed by a large number of people—in shocking numbers. In 1988, 17 percent of Americans said they never attended religious services. By 2021, that number had almost doubled—to 31 percent.

    At this point, you might be wondering if I've started wearing vestments and calling myself "Reverend Phil" instead of "Dr. Phil." Nope, I'm not here to proselytize (although maybe I'm being a little preachy), but as I suggest in the title, I am fighting for the collective soul of our country. When I say collective soul, I mean our character, free will, reason, feeling, consciousness, perception, thinking, and our memory of what this country has been and how we got to be that shining city on a hill. In an earlier chapter, I talk about the collective personality in the example of a jury, and the collective personality of the community, the state, and our nation. At the core is our collective *soul.* When we allow revisionist historians to overwrite that which has been imprinted on the soul of our country, everything starts to unravel. We can't just forget who we are. In simpler terms, we have to "dance with who brung us." So, I'm here on a different calling, which is to inspire you to stand strong for our soul and sanity—what this country has been and part of what *you* have been, as well as what it can be, so that we do not let it slip away. This is as much a spiritual battle as it is any other kind.

According to a *Frontiers in Psychology* study, spirituality is directly associated with psychological well-being.[3] Adults who attended religious services at least monthly as adolescents were more likely to be happy as adults.[4] And actively religious adults smoke and drink less—and even though they don't necessarily exercise more—they live longer and cope with stress better.[5]

We are in a mental health crisis in this country right now, and one of the solutions is staring us in the face!

One of the things I've noticed, and maybe you have too, is that very few people attend church alone. It has a way of bringing together families and communities. It creates an opportunity to come together in a shared moment of reverence, a social interaction, which science tells us strengthens social bonds. In a divided society, a communal worshiping experience helps create unity and social cohesion.[6] This has major implications, because the absence of social cohesion is one of the key preconditions for conflict and violence.

The fundamental values underpinning the major religions also teach people how to be good members of society. The Ten Commandments may be the most widely known set of rules for moral behavior in existence.[7] Also known as the Decalogue, these ten rules form the foundation of Christianity, Judaism, and Islam. And there's a reason these ten things aren't mere suggestions but are commandments: because society stops functioning if we don't follow them.

We are not the first people to have decided we don't have to follow the rules and, instead, can just make them up as we go along. The prophet Samuel's very last words in the book of Judges was to observe that the people of Israel had fallen into the "my personal truth" mode, as we now have, and lament that "every man did that which was right in his own eyes."[8] Rules had gone out the window. The people, back then in Samuel's day, were making up the rules that were "right in their own eyes." The moral couldn't be clearer: society suffered mightily because of it. So will we.

After all, bringing in the wisdom of Proverbs: "The way of a fool is right in his own eyes."[9]

One problem is that we aren't just disobeying these rules. We are violating them with *pride* rather than shame.

Take "envy," for example. Not coveting what other people have is one of the ten rules—Thou Shalt Not Covet. You may wonder, how did a rule against being envious make the top ten? Aren't there worse things? Apparently not, because envy gets equal billing in the Ten Commandments with murder and lying. Yet we are not only openly envious: envy has become institutionalized as a political tactic. In fact, when you look at the debate around income inequality, if you were to argue that we actually have too much income equality (as I do in our section about rewarding hard work, skill, and knowledge), then hold on to your hat, because you're going to come in for some criticism.

So, we've embraced envy and we attack those who argue against envy despite current learning that has exposed the corrosive and destructive effects envy has on society.

Renowned sociologist Helmut Schoeck, who wrote an entire book on envy, described it this way: "No society can exist in which envy [is] raised to the status of a normative virtue. . . ." But that is precisely what we are doing. That's really what the debate about "income inequality" is all about. It's not a call to arms, it's a call to envy. "These people have more, and we should have some of that."

Homicide is rampant in our country, especially compared to other developed countries such as Germany, France, Italy, Japan, Spain, and the United Kingdom, who all have murder rates a fraction of ours.[10] But at least we don't criticize those who don't commit homicide.

We have turned that particular commandment against envy on its head by making envy a normative virtue. No society can survive doing that. Perhaps a little time in the pews of our churches would help us be a better society and, in the process, help save our country.

Or consider the commandment against stealing, which is today being violated with impunity.

As I'm writing this, Target has reported that theft could be costing them upward of $1 billion, and that retailers lost up to $80 billion in theft in 2022—up by $13 billion in one year. Theft is running so rampant in some areas that retailers from Target to CVS and Whole Foods are being forced to close stores.[11]

In New York, research has shown that nearly one-third of all arrests for shoplifting—we're talking about 6,000 arrests—involved the same 327 people.[12] But they can afford to keep doing it and keep getting arrested, because punishment is nonexistent. And while these thefts may be called property crimes, the truth is that a smash-and-grab is a violent crime. It's scary, it's intimidating, and it can drive a small enterprise out of business.

You hear a lot about the costs of incarceration—the cost of imprisoning people, and the fact that they are rarely rehabilitated. But what about the costs of *decarceration*—the costs of allowing people to be out on the street who, based on their criminal history, shouldn't be?

The National Retail Federation conducts an annual survey regarding "shrink," which is a term that includes projected inventory losses from shoplifting and employee theft, as well as some other factors. In 2021, "shrink" hit $94.5 billion, a 53 percent jump from 2019!

What in the world is making this okay in people's minds? Yes, a lot of this is organized crime. But a lot is people just deciding to take what isn't theirs, comfortable in the fact they are highly unlikely to be prosecuted even if arrested. They have just made up their own rules, unconcerned about having broken God's commandments or the law of the land. They operate by their own rule of "Take what you want," which has only taken hold because they have learned that there's no punishment for theft. They feel perfectly entitled to what they are taking. The woke mob has supported the mindset that everyone is entitled to an equal outcome. If they don't have that standard of living they believe they're entitled to, just take the difference. They didn't earn it, they didn't work for it, they just claimed it. And no one is punished.

Actually, that's not quite true—everyone who chooses not to steal is the one being punished, by higher prices and closing stores. Those of us who don't steal pay for those who do. It is that simple.

When people are stealing at a rate that causes stores to just throw up their hands and close because the cost of loss due to theft is too high to survive (and they are doing this by the dozens), something has gone seriously askew. The moral compass has lost its true north.

Fixing the compass begins with a return to the practice and expression of faith in God, which offers a good reminder of core values and an effective means to strengthening family, because, as I said, most people attend church as a family. It's a means to community because it fosters a sense of involvement, engagement, and belonging. And it's a conduit for receiving a moral education and understanding and willfully obeying society's rules. But when you lose faith or drift away from the practice of it, you actually lose all of those things too.

Speaking of the Ten Commandments, I have a pop quiz for you. What are the first two?

If you're like most people, your mind probably went to one of the "legal" ones—thou shalt not kill, or steal, or commit adultery, or covet.

But the first two of the Ten Commandments speak to something that may not seem immediately relevant today, but that I would argue are the *most* relevant right now.

viction? And how does that routine practice of your faith improve your life and relationships?

In the poll I conducted of my viewers, I asked how often they attend an organized religious service. Given the particular sample I polled, one might assume that we'd see far more "weekly or more" answers. But in fact, less than 30 percent said "weekly or more," and nearly 40 percent of respondents said they never attend. I think this, together with the evidence and examples we've talked about in this chapter, indicates there is a deep need for a spiritual wake-up call in this country.

POLL RESPONSE

How often do you attend organized religious service?

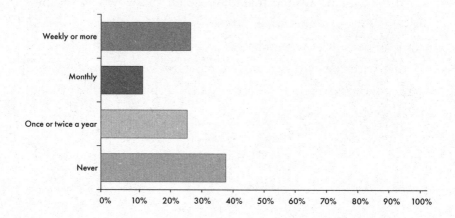

Far be it from me to criticize those who, for their own reasons, do not attend church services. But as a psychologist who recognizes the therapeutic benefits of church attendance, I'd submit to you that maybe it is time for all of us to rethink and clearly define our view of faith. Rethink the model you are providing as a parent. Rethink the value of spending some time with God in a sacred space. Rethink the benefits of introspection about our own shortcomings as an important step toward doing better. And if you are dwelling on those things, think about the fact that there is always a really good seat waiting for you in church, along with a wealth of opportunities to love your neighbors.

CHAPTER 17

Science Is Under Attack

POLL QUESTION

Who should have access to gender transition–related medical services?

- ☐ Adults only
- ☐ Adults and under 18 with parental permission
- ☐ Under 18 without parental permission
- ☐ No one

I've noted several times so far that it often feels like science is under attack.

Let me use an issue that's in the headlines to explain what I mean.

Many parents and others object to medical doctors providing what the transgender community and a portion of the medical community refer to as "gender-affirming care," for fear that it is nothing more than surgical mutilation or hormonal destruction of natural development. Some medical organizations have expressed concerns about "gender-affirming care," especially for minors. However, some of the larger and most powerful medical associations in the country, like the American Academy of Pediatrics, the American Medical Association, the World Health Organization, and the Endocrine Society (which deals directly with hormonal issues), recommend that transgender youth be able to access this kind of health care.

Having reviewed the literature concerning the medical transition of prepubescent children, I am nothing short of shocked that the leadership of these professional organizations has endorsed these procedures. They must either be advancing their own personal agendas or have caved to the Tyranny of the Fringe. Either way, I don't think history will be kind to them. I conclude this because I know of no other instance in which the medical profession has proceeded with so little or no evidence as to whether these hormonal treatments are safe over the long term or whether surgery will have long-term detrimental effects. The surgical procedures on pubescent children are certainly not reversible.

According to the American Civil Liberties Union at the time of this writing, more than thirty-four states have bans or restrictions proposed or in place, and there are over one hundred pieces of legislation moving through statehouses to stop "gender-affirming care" primarily for children under eighteen. The state attorneys general allege these major medical organizations are assuming their supportive positions absent sufficient empirical evidence. The medical organizations are referring to the "gender-affirming" procedures as "evidence based." This is misleading because it primarily refers to psychological impact and not the physical impact of what many consider radical treatment—one that can be administered without proper screening and parental involvement.

In some states such as Oregon, fifteen- and sixteen-year-olds can walk into a medical establishment without parental consent and receive hormone treatments. Similarly in Oregon, teens as young as seventeen and eighteen can also get "top surgery," which is a double mastectomy—and they can do it with no parental permission.

"Gender-affirming care" can involve children getting puberty blockers not approved by the Food and Drug Administration. This includes Lupron, a drug originally used to chemically castrate chronic sex offenders.

It's important to note that gender dysphoria, listed in the American Psychiatric Association's *Diagnostic and Statistical Manual of Mental Disorders*, fifth edition (DSM-5), is very real and should not be trivialized. It occurs at a rate of about one in ten thousand. It mostly affects boys with an onset around two to four years of age. Most will grow out of it over time if left alone. So, how can these medical professions accept self-diagnoses, particularly from teenage girls? And by the way, most of these girls now claiming gender dysphoria had no history of dysphoria as a child, which would be typical, a diagnostic "red flag."

I've read studies where some in the medical community poohpooh the idea of "social contagion." But I think that's exactly what we're seeing when it comes to girls and gender dysphoria. One data point that I found striking was in a study out of the United Kingdom, where the Gender Identity Development Service found a 4,400 percent increase in the number of girls who wanted to change their sex. And these were girls who had no previous history of feeling distressed about their biological sex.

What's interesting here is that if this increase were due to more awareness and acceptance of people who feel—as some very seriously and legitimately do—that they are trapped in the wrong body, we would see similar increases across other demographics, like middle-aged women, or men.

But they didn't see that.

So something else must be at play.

Could it be that these girls were getting hooked on an idea after being exposed to it on social media or within their peer group? We've seen that happen with girls and eating disorders.

I submit to you that the media focus, headlines, and social media are powerful drivers, and to ignore those factors is foolish and unprofessional. Citing that research is *not* "hate speech," it is just reporting the facts.

Doctors argue they must rush in because of high suicide rates among those "feeling trapped" in the wrong body. Their attitude is

"Get them out of this gender prison, stat!" as if that will make all of the associated problems go away. But any evidence showing that puberty blockers ameliorate suicidality or even improve mental health is scant and not supported in the real world. The medical groups' support for transitioning—especially with young children—is scientifically inexplicable to me. The "patients" who receive "gender-affirming care" are left underdeveloped compared to their peers in terms of sex organs, and are often disrupted developmentally in other ways. Yes, there may be an initial euphoria that one of the mental and emotional "conflicts" in their life is being resolved. But these treatments offer a dramatic change, not a cure-all. All the comorbidities, the propensity for self-harm, the propensity for substance abuse—if those aren't resolved first, two bad things can happen: The first is that a young person can go into this process while they aren't able to look clearly at their gender dysphoria. The second is that they may expect a cure-all only to find the underlying (or connected) issues still unresolved. Even in a different body, you are still *you*. I hark back to the Hippocratic Oath, taken by physicians, in which they pledge to "first do no harm."

I clearly disagree with these medical organizations on many different levels. However, I am including the fact that they endorse transitioning certain young children because it is factual even if, in my opinion, misguided.

With regard to determining the sex of a newborn and how that decision is made, the vast majority of the population believe sex is *defined* at birth and before by external genitalia and confirmed by their chromosomes.

If I understand correctly, the transgender community now holds that sex is only *assigned*, not *defined* at birth based on external genitalia. They further believe that a person can transition their sex and not just their gender. In the not-too-distant past, transgender women did not claim to *actually be women*; they found comfort and peace presenting to the world as feminine and living as transgender females. Today the activists, and I believe an unknown portion of the transgender community, now claim they *are* women. My research team and I have had to dig really deep to find a consensus opinion on what the transgender community holds to now be true about sex. What gets "shouted" is that transgender women *are* women, and that sex is nonbinary.

Even though I don't believe anyone can just rewrite biological history, I have made a good-faith effort to describe that with which I believe members of the transgender community would agree. If I have missed any nuance, it is unintentional, and I recommend visiting the site of the LGBTQ advocacy organization GLAAD, particularly the "Glossary" sections, to gather your own information and look up my many references. GLAAD is a respected organization, and GLAAD .org is a very user-friendly site.

As of this writing, Bud Light, a popular beer, saw their sales slump by 26 percent and lost their position as the number one beer sold in America after working with a transgender social media influencer.[1] Target retail stores are reported to have lost $12 billion–$14 billion in market value for aggressively displaying "tuck friendly" swimwear in their stores nationwide as part of their "Pride collection."

There seems to be a clear disconnect between the transgender community's beliefs and agendas and what mainstream America is comfortable with accepting or endorsing. But hey, President Biden stepped up and said, "Transgender Americans shape our nation's soul." Certainly, transgender Americans—like every American—have the right to live their lives, speak, gather, and worship freely. Certainly, we should all treat each other with dignity and respect, and work to find common ground. But when I heard that statement, I thought that the trans community might *want* to shape our nation's soul, but no, Mr. President, I think an awful lot of Americans might not totally agree with your statement. That doesn't make them "haters." I just don't think they would go quite that far, and I think a balanced assessment would reveal that many think the transgender community, or at least their activists, are pushing their agenda and their fight for their rights to the point that it is infringing on other Americans' rights.

Again, I'm focusing on this issue because it is one of many where one group's beliefs and agenda are pushing Americans beyond what they are comfortable with accepting or endorsing, and damaging its own agenda in the process.

A current example is seen in the case of transgender athletes, particularly transgender women (men who transition to become women) competing against biological women and in many cases dominating the competition. A recent poll found that even as more Americans know someone who is transgender, fewer Americans think that transgender athletes should be able to compete as anything other than their birth gender identity, rather than their assumed gender identity.[2]

> **I'm focusing on this issue because it is one of many where one group's beliefs and agenda are pushing Americans beyond what they are comfortable with accepting or endorsing, and damaging its own agenda in the process.**

I get it. That doesn't make people who feel that way haters. You don't need to hear many stories like the high school women's volleyball player who was concussed by her transgender opponent to feel uncomfortable with this.[3] Even President Biden "seems" to get it—that's why he decided to allow universities and K–12 schools the ability to limit the participation of transgender students if including them would get in the way of competitive fairness or increase the risk of injury.[4]

But this isn't really a matter of "if." Dr. Carole Hooven, the former codirector of Undergraduate Studies of Human Evolutionary Biology at Harvard University, describes testosterone's massive influence on men's greater size, strength, and speed in her book *T: The Story of Testosterone, the Hormone That Dominates and Divides Us.*

She cites extensive research that addresses the question of

whether the typical male advantage in most sports—from about 10 to 50 percent—is lost when males take testosterone-blocking drugs ("blockers") to suppress their naturally high testosterone levels as part of a gender transition. If scientific research demonstrated that using blockers meant a loss of that advantage over women, then perhaps it would be fair for transgender women (who block or reduce their testosterone) to compete in the female sports category.

Hooven's analysis of the relevant research, including papers like a highly influential one from 2021 by Emma Hilton and Tommy Lundberg, "Transgender Women in the Female Category of Sport: Perspectives on Testosterone Suppression and Performance Advantage," demonstrates that male advantage is not lost.

In other words, transgender women who went through male puberty retain a significant advantage in strength, speed, and power over women. And this is the conclusion reached by all the relevant research. In fact, suppressing testosterone for up to three years has been shown to have a minimal impact on strength and muscle mass, not to mention no effect on other traits like bone density, height, and lung capacity, which all provide a sporting advantage.

So to the extent that fairness is based on scientific and biological reality, Hooven concludes that it's just not fair for transgender women to compete against biological females. Her view is not driven by any animosity toward transgender people, but instead by scientific evidence and biology. Having male-bodied people, particularly those who have experienced the benefits of male puberty, compete in the female category is not fair and never will be, regardless of what measures are taken to blunt those pubertal benefits, like enhanced muscle mass, present before transitioning. She offers no political or psychosocial opinion; she just reports the scientific findings. She is not a hater.

She's reached this conclusion because, as an evolutionary biologist and expert on testosterone, she understands that the effect of high testosterone on boys and men is to equip them with the traits that have benefited them reproductively over human evolutionary history. And testosterone starts doing its job in very early development, when the male fetus starts producing levels of testosterone that are several times higher than fetal female levels, about as high as they will be again in male puberty!

The result is that after male puberty, despite hormone therapy such as testosterone blockers (T blockers), most biological makeup won't change. Organ size, height, bone density, and lung capacity are already established and it's impossible to fully reverse those attributes. Scientific analysis of human biology confirms:

- ➤ Males carry 15 times the amount of testosterone as females.

- ➤ Males carry 11 percent more hemoglobin, which carries oxygen to the blood. With more oxygen in blood, organs function at higher efficiency, which directly affects athletes' performance. This is why "blood doping" is a way for athletes to cheat—they're finding ways for their blood to carry more oxygen. (After prolonged T blockers, hemoglobin levels are more similar to female levels, but everything else remains the same.)

- ➤ Men have 45 percent more lean body mass and 30–50 percent less body fat than women. After 3 years of T blockers, muscle mass only drops an average of 3–5 percent, and body fat increases somewhat.

- ➤ Males have advantages in: height, wingspan, bone strength, heart capacity, and lung volume.

- ➤ Males have a 40 percent upper-body-strength advantage, and even after T blockers it only drops by 10 percent.

Overall, it is not a close call. Transgender women are still stronger, taller, and leaner than biological females, in addition to the other anatomical advantages at play (bone density, heart and lung size, cellular composition).

Males' performance advantages range from:

➤ A 10 percent advantage in swimming and running, races that often come down to hundredths or even thousandths of a second (Ten percent could be twelve seconds in a two-minute race!)

➤ 50 percent or more in throwing speed

➤ 30 percent greater strength in weight lifting

➤ 60 percent higher grip strength

To further empirically support the answer that it simply is not fair for transgender girls or women to compete against biological girls or women, a study published by Duke University Law School's Center for Sports Law and Policy reports that in the single year of 2017, Olympic, world, and US women's track and field champion Tori Bowie's 100-meters lifetime best time of 10.78 seconds has been beaten 15,000 times by men and boys.

Similarly, Olympic, world, and US champion Allyson Felix's lifetime best time of 49.26 seconds in the 400 meters was beaten 15,000 times by men and boys around the world as well.

Looking at those results in the context of Dr. Hooven's conclusion that even with T blockers you cannot erase enough of the male advantages to come even close to leveling the competitive playing field, it is simply not fair for transgender women to compete against biological women. (The Duke Law article poses several well-stated questions and there is a link to it in the endnotes.)[5]

Transgender athletes should not be denied the joy of athletics, the camaraderie of participating, or the thrill of competition. But they should have their own category or classification. That is not discriminatory to suggest. Many sports have always been divided by sex, weight stratification, experience, or skill level. This would just be one more classification or division. It has worked well for a long time and is a system that should not be scrapped because one activist group believes that two groups of people are the same when biologically, empirically, fundamentally, they are not. The playing field should be about fair play.

Still, people are uncomfortable speaking out about transgender issues in sports, schools, or life in general. But as we see with Target and Bud Light, they are speaking with their wallets. It takes a lot of people changing spending habits to have that big an impact on national brands, and that's why I think that's pretty good evidence that I'm right when I say people feel more strongly than they are comfortable saying out loud.

Would all of those people have spoken up and risked being labeled transphobic? Obviously not. But when they could make their position known anonymously by altering their spending habits, it spoke volumes. It also suggests that mainstream America is not nearly as aligned with the agenda as corporate America mistakenly reads them to be.

POLL RESPONSE

Who should have access to gender transition–related medical services?

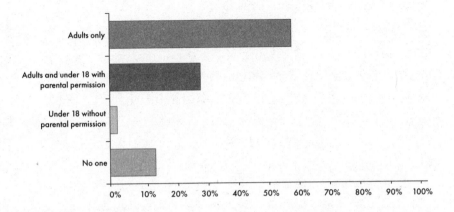

Now, I've let you know how I feel about this. I'm not a physician so you have to take my opinion about these medical services with a grain of salt. And even though we disagree, I included the fact that major medical organizations disagree with me. Now, who has the most credibility: me, a nonmedical professional, or these major medical organizations? That's why I included them. They are credible medical organizations. And even acknowledging that, I still stand by my position that they don't have the empirical evidence that it does not create long-term harm. But they disagree, and they have signed off on this. I don't think history will be kind to them. These are the same medical associations that suggested smoking cigarettes to relieve your anxiety in the past. They don't always get it right, and I think this is one where they're not getting it right. You make up your own mind.

PART FOUR

The Ten Working Principles
for a Healthy Society

As I said in the introduction, take a step back and look at where we are as a country. We've gotten rid of one of the most important American traits, self-determination, and replaced it with victimization. We've gotten rid of conversation and replaced it with cancellation. We've gone from courageous to coddled. We've decided to celebrate intent, rather than outcomes. And we're all paying the price for it, spiritually, emotionally, and financially.

We will never, ever whine our way to success (even though social media allows some people to try).

We will never blame our way to fulfillment.

The government will never be able to "entitle" us to self-actualization.

Government cannot give us that pride of accomplishment that only comes from hard work and observing oneself persevere.

There is no victory in "victimhood."

We seem to have forgotten the difference between a "hand up," which we can all use from time to time, and a handout, which starts as a Band-Aid and slowly becomes a crutch that if you lean on long enough, you can forget how to walk.

There will never be a sustainable "equality of outcome" no matter how popular the concept. There may never be full equality of opportunity, for that matter.

If you believe in individualism, you have to accept individual differences.

We can work on creating equities as a society, but it really is true that you can only "help those that help themselves."

I've been watching this decline for a long time, like a snowball rolling down a hill, getting bigger, picking up speed. Which means it will take more to stop it today than it did yesterday, and more to stop it tomorrow than it does today. Put something small in front of it, and it'll just swallow it up and keep rolling.

So, I'm proposing we put something big in front of it. Ten things, actually. Ten principles that we need to live and operate by, in order to stop the slide and reclaim success for your life, your community, your state, and *our* country.

I call them my ten working principles for a healthy society. I'll list them for you right here, and then explain them—with evidence and examples—in the following chapters.

Principle #1: Be Who You Are on Purpose

Principle #2: Focus on Solving Problems Rather Than Winning Arguments

Principle #3: Don't Reward Bad Behavior or Support Conduct You Do Not Value

Principle #4: Measure All Actions Based on Results, and All Thoughts Based on Rationality

Principle #5: Consciously Choose Which Voices in Your Life Deserve the Most Attention

Principle #6: Do Not Stay Silent So Others Can Remain Comfortable

Principle #7: Actively Live and Support a Meritocracy

Principle #8: Identify and Build Your Consequential Knowledge

Principle #9: Work Hard to Understand the Way Others See Things

Principle #10: Treat Yourself and Others with Dignity and Respect

If we adhere to these ten working principles—these ten guides—a lot of things, in your life and in our country, are going to start looking very different.

PRINCIPLE #1

Be Who You Are on Purpose

POLL QUESTION

How often do you let other people's negative opinions of you
or your beliefs affect/impact you?

☐ Always

☐ Very often

☐ Sometimes

☐ Never

You've made it this far in this book, and I'm happy about that.

More importantly, I hope you're happy about that.

I hope you're finding it clarifying and helpful.

But what if you're one of just a small handful of people who are reading this book, when my publisher and I expected hundreds of thousands or even millions?

What if this book is a flop of massive proportions?

You know what? I admit I would be surprised and very disappointed, but nonetheless that would be totally "on me." No one else, just me.

I own the decisions I've made and the path I've taken. Or, rather, the paths. That's how I've lived my life from a very young age, actually. Once married to Robin I've always discussed major decisions and made them in partnership with her, of course, but when those decisions even after discussion were left to me to decide or act upon personally, I *owned* them. Career-wise I have had three main phases in my life—and at each phase, I left a very successful and comfortable circumstance to move into a different one.

For years, as a practicing clinical psychologist, I had a very successful private practice. For a long time, that was my dream. In fact, it exceeded any idea I ever had of what it could look like. I could have kept that practice going and rode that horse for my entire life, into a happy retirement sunset.

But then I felt like I had done all I was meant to do and became extremely passionate about evolving a very technical trial science company in the high-stakes litigation arena. With Robin's support and a lot of amazing support from people who are among my closest and best friends to this day, we built that into what I believe was the most successful and effective trial science company in America. I could have gotten comfortable there and rode that horse into retirement. But there came a point when I felt like after many years that I had "climbed that mountain." I had done just about every category of litigation there was to do, many times over.

Then came the challenge and opportunity of entering the broadcasting world. I'm sure some might look at me and say, "What is the deal, you can't stand success? Are you insane?" It may have looked that way because I walked away from that hard-earned pinnacle and took on the extremely high-risk endeavor of launching my own television show. Again, with a lot and I do mean a lot of help (Oprah) and over twenty-five years, I built one of the most popular TV shows in America. After twenty-one successful seasons and no longer being a "spring chicken," I certainly could have justified riding that horse as long as I wanted until retirement. But once again I decided to walk away from "legacy level" success and take on a new challenge.

Now you could argue that maybe I've got adult attention-deficit disorder. Or you could say that I'm playing career Russian roulette, and one of these days there's going to be one in the chamber. But I prefer to see it as an extreme version of practicing what I preach. And what I've been preaching my whole life is the gospel of being who you are on purpose. I am unwilling to give my power away by being controlled by what other people think or *expect* me to do. I don't care how what I do or don't do looks to other people. I don't care if it makes consensual sense. I have to be who I am *on purpose.* I said earlier I had been that way from a young age. Maybe that is one unintended consequence of being the child of an alcoholic father.

> **I don't care how what I do or don't do looks to other people. I don't care if it makes consensual sense. I have to be who I am *on purpose.***

In chapter 1, I told you to give yourself permission to consciously acknowledge who you choose to be, who you are, what you are making happen around you, and what you are allowing to happen around you. Own you!

In chapter 6, I reminded you that everywhere we turn, people, companies, political parties, and media platforms are trying to influence you, own you, pull you left, pull you right, pull you into their camp, recruit you into their way of seeing the world. Protest this! Join that!

In chapter 15, I talked about how important being who you are on purpose matters to your family, so that you model the behaviors you want to see passed down through the generations.

The reason this theme keeps showing up is that being who you are on purpose matters.

It matters for you, because there's nothing sadder than waking up to realize that you sleepwalked into a life you didn't choose. That you went the way the river was taking you. That you didn't make choices, you made concessions. You didn't captain your life, you capitulated to it.

But it also matters for us—all of us. I've made clear that we've lost our way in this country. And the only way to find our way back is for us—all of us—to stop living our lives according to some agenda that's being presented to us, and instead setting the priorities we want to set, taking the positions we want to take, and doing these things consciously, on purpose. This life you are living is no dress rehearsal. This is it. You need to star in your own life. If you don't, who will? I just want you to be sure you make your life count, you make your voice heard, you make your beliefs felt. You don't have to be an activist unless that is who you are. You just want to be you and do it with intention, do it on purpose.

Our country's soul and sanity depend on it.

POLL RESPONSE

How often do you let other people's negative opinions of you or your beliefs affect/impact you?

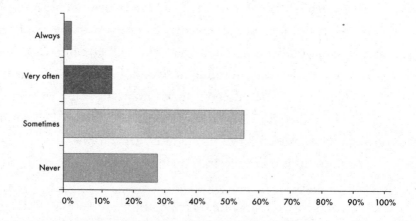

Focus on Solving Problems Rather Than Winning Arguments

POLL QUESTION

If you're being totally honest with yourself, when you are in conflict with someone you care about, how often are you focused on being right/winning the argument, rather than resolving the problem?

☐ Always
☐ Very often
☐ Sometimes
☐ Never

I may surprise you in the next several pages with some of the things I'm about to say. You may need to read it, think about it some, and come back to it again because it may violate your beliefs and sound somewhat paranoid. I don't think it is, but I'll let you decide.

I submit that some of the people we have designated to lead the charge on solving some of our biggest problems are going through the motions, and in fact have absolutely no desire whatsoever to solve the problem to which they have been assigned. In fact, solving the problem may put them out of a job.

Who Doesn't Want to Solve Problems?

That's right, I believe many of the people who achieve their positions of power by pledging to solve problems don't actually have any interest in doing that.

Their goal is to get reelected, not to solve your problem. If they are in the private sector, their goal is to keep and grow their jobs, and they aren't going to do that by eliminating the reason they were hired in the first place.

In fact, by one measure, politicians spend more of their time in office fundraising than legislating. And you know what helps you raise money—*not* solving problems.

Because an unsolved problem leads to outrage, the emotional buy-in that leads to both fundraising dollars and votes.

Democrats and Republicans *need* an immigration crisis.

Israeli and Palestinian politicians need the permanent conflict (even if their constituents don't) so they can fire up popular passion and stay in office.

Forever problems lead to forever fundraising and forever jobs.

Nobody willingly puts themselves out of business.

That's why it was a big deal back in 2006 when the Bill & Melinda Gates Foundation—the biggest foundation in the world—announced that it would close up shop within fifty years of the death of its three trustees.

Here's how they described it: "The decision to focus all of our resources in this century underscores our optimism for making huge progress and for making sure that we do as much as possible, as soon as possible, on the comparatively narrow set of issues we've chosen to focus on."[1]

So, they're saying: If you're looking to us to provide forever jobs, you're out of luck. If you're a charity looking for us to fund you forever, you're out of luck. We started this thing in order to solve some problems. And we're going to spend every dime we have trying to do that. Because our interest isn't in prolonging a problem. Our interest is in solving a problem.

Right now, we have so many issues in America that could have been settled on a reasonable middle ground marked by tolerance and compromise. But our "leaders"—as cynical as it may sound—just can't afford financially, egotistically, or socially to have peace breaking out!

The difference in the two approaches—between solving a problem and winning an argument—is like daylight and darkness. If someone enters a situation focused on winning an argument, their focus is on beating *you*.

Here's how you'll spot that.

Their conduct will be marked by a lack of understanding, intolerance, even hostility. They will try to shut down your contentions and assertions rather than respectfully hearing them out and allowing them to be heard by others. They will try to trap you in contradictions. They will make you feel foolish. At some point, they'll stop trying to shut down your points and start trying to shut down *you*. They've now made it personal, because you've had the audacity to disagree. It's not long before any hope for sparking new ideas born out of collaboration is lost—it's no longer on the table. There's no chance for creativity, and lots of missed opportunities for growth and development. Positions harden, battle lines are drawn, and the result is stagnation and little, if any, learning.

> **Never forget that when you define any relationship in a "win-lose" framework, that means there is going to be a *winner* and a *loser*. But in truth, everyone has lost along the way.**

Never forget that when you define any relationship in a "win-lose" framework, that means there is going to be a *winner* and a *loser*. But in truth, everyone has lost along the way. When you lost, how did it feel? Did you like it? Of course not. I submit to you that every "win-lose" scenario is really a "lose-lose" scenario. A saying frequently attributed to Samuel Butler's satirical poem *Hudibras* from the 1600s resonates: "A man convinced against his will is of the same opinion still."

By contrast, you can spot if someone is genuinely interested in solving a problem rather than just winning an argument. They will immediately engage in a *collaborative* process rather than being a dictatorial fighter. They will welcome your point of view and listen, listen, and actively listen. That means they'll be able to reflect your position back to you authentically. They might say something like "So, if I'm hearing you correctly, your position is . . ." and then give a fair statement of it. And then say, "And you feel that way because . . ." and give a fair statement of your motivations.

They may also suggest or respond openly when you suggest that both sides work to identify everything you can agree on *before* focusing areas of difference in an effort to build some common ground and narrow the scope and number of the problems to be solved.

I tell the people I teach to not only find out what the person across the table wants, but why they want it. Everybody has a different kind of currency. You may find out there are some concessions that could be a small give to you, but a big get to them. A 10 on their list might be a 2 on yours!

For example, in one of my contract negotiations, there was one item that was very important to me, and so I raised it. Turns out it was totally unimportant to CBS. We never would have figured that out if we hadn't worked out why each of us wanted what we wanted.

In successful attempts to solve problems, you will hear statements such as "What if we tried to come up with some first steps we could both live with?" Or "Is it possible we could table a few of these stubborn issues and make some progress on a few of the areas that seem really important to you?" They will ask open-ended questions, not just a "yes" or "no." You may hear them thank you for helping them grasp the what and why of your position. Statements like this won't be a concession that they agree, but that they have learned something.

A simple turn of phrase such as "I need your help in coming up with a solution that can solve at least a part of this problem, so thank you for working with me on this" or "Together surely we can make some progress" is incredibly powerful in the problem-solving process, because people want to feel like they are part of a team. They are much less likely to criticize a plan they have some authorship in writing. After all, you don't want to tip over a boat that you're in!

And when you've concluded a negotiation or a discussion with your children, or spouse, or involving a work or community situation, do an autopsy on your approach. How would you categorize your posture? What worked? What didn't?

Once an agreement is made, and this is key, too, *move forward*.

Once the deal is done, get to work making the best of it. Successes build on themselves. When you work through problems with people, they build an expectation that the next problems will be worked through as well, and before long, you have a winning relationship.

I want to tell you the story of a guy named Dr. Raj Shah. Dr. Shah is the president of the Rockefeller Foundation, but under President Barack Obama he was in charge of an agency called USAID, which hands out foreign aid to people in other countries.

In 2010, Republicans proposed a bill to cut funding for foreign aid and development. Dr. Shah was deeply worried, because these cuts would dramatically reduce his ability to deliver food aid. And because he's a data guy, he ran an analysis of what the budget cuts would mean to his goals of helping America save lives all over the world. The analysis showed that the cuts would lead to 70,000 children dying. According to his math, 30,000 would die from a cut in programs to prevent malaria; 24,000 would die because they wouldn't get childhood immunizations; and another 16,000 would die at birth from lack of nutrition and other causes.

What did he do with that analysis? He went public with it. And you can guess what happened. Everyone started running around and screaming, more or less. Democrats started screaming that finally, finally, someone had the cojones to show just what heartless scrooges Republicans were being. Republicans were screaming mad that they had just been called mass murderers for suggesting that maybe our government should live within its means.

Dr. Shah had a choice. A lot of his fans—a lot of the people he worked for—loved seeing him stick it to Republicans. He could go on MSNBC and CNN to his heart's content and tell everyone how terrible Republicans were. He could try to win an argument. After all, he believed in his numbers. Or he could try to solve a problem.

Here's how he described his choice: "I saw two paths forward. I could double down, becoming a partisan warrior who throws heat on Twitter and cable news. Or I could make amends and attempt to build better and deeper relationships with Republicans and others, connections that were not merely transactional or technocratic, but based on shared values and common interests."

So that's what he did—he tried to solve the problem. He apologized to the folks he had offended. There's a saying that a man never stands taller than when he stoops to kiss an ass—by that measure, Dr. Shah stood pretty tall for a while. And then he worked to actually get to know the folks who wanted to cut his funding. He met with them, traveled with them, prayed with them. He got to understand their values and concerns, and they got to understand his passion.

A couple of months later, when the budget was finalized, not only was his funding not cut, it was actually *increased*. That wouldn't have happened if Dr. Shah was screaming his head off on cable news. It happened because he chose to solve a problem rather than win an argument.

Ask the Right Questions

Albert Einstein is believed to have said that if he had an hour to save the world, he would spend fifty-five minutes defining the problem. Charles Kettering, who was the head of innovation at General Motors, said that a problem well stated is half-solved. Accurately describing the problems we face will go a long way toward solutions to those problems, and that means asking the right question.

Look at one of our hottest hot-button issues, immigration. The question is not should we build a wall and keep everyone out—we know that's not working. It's not should we open our hearts and borders and let everyone in—we know that's not working either. It's "What do we actually need as a country? What does a good outcome look like?"

Right now in Texas, where I live, birth rates are falling faster than they are in the rest of the nation. The Federal Reserve Bank of Dallas predicts that this will slow economic growth, and that fewer young workers, in particular, will reduce productivity.[2] In short, Texas needs immigrants. So, to me, a better question is "How can we welcome immigrants who will work hard, embrace America, and not commit crimes?" That, to me, is a much better question than the same ones we've been asking for decades, which may keep people on both the left and right in office but haven't done a darn thing to solve the problem.

Or take an even hotter hot-button issue: school shooters and mass shooters. Notice that here I'm saying "shooters" and not "shootings." I want to focus on a problem that is manageable, a problem open to solutions. I understand why some people want to have a gun debate. But that debate hasn't gotten us anywhere, and meanwhile we live in a country of 330 million people and 400 million guns, where mass shootings have become more frequent and deadlier than ever. Even if no more guns were manufactured starting today, there would still be millions of guns around for hundred of years—and we need to impact this problem now. I have been intensively studying school shooters and have concluded that we know a lot more about shooters in general, and school shooters in particular, than we are using to generate solutions. We can do significantly more to impact the frequency of these tragic school shootings than we are doing.

I've spent a lot of time talking to Dr. Jillian Peterson, who is a psychologist, and Dr. James Densley, who is a sociologist. They run an organization called the Violence Project and have developed an integrated, interdisciplinary understanding of violence and a holistic approach to addressing it. They are, in my opinion, the top experts in the world when it comes to researching and understanding why these shooters do what they do and how to use that information.

Peterson and Densley have identified a series of traits that mass shooters have in common and, as a subset, those who target schools.

Here is what we know about who does this:

Age/Race/Gender: 16–19/White/Male

Family history: Early and unresolved childhood trauma

Family Profile: One or both parents dysfunctional (abusive, drugs, prison history, psychological problems)

Psychological Adjustment: Observable mental health problems when most shootings happen

Social Adjustment: Marginalized. Likely experienced some type of rejection in recent past

Leakage: 90+ percent tell at least one person what they are going to do and when they are going to do it. Almost 70 percent of the time they tell two or more people, and oftentimes one of the people they tell is in law enforcement.

Target: 90+ percent target a school they either attend or previously attended

Guns: 90 percent get the guns by stealing them from home or friends where they are *unlocked*

Motive: Twofold: revenge for transgressions real or imagined and to die by violent suicide

Time of the year: High-stress times in the school year, like right before or after a break. Strangely enough, shootings also occur disproportionately on the twentieth of any given month.

A Strategy for Safety

When I say we know more than we are using, the checklist above is evidence of what we know but does not mean we can predict who will become a school shooter and who won't. What it does suggest is how schools can become more vigilant and take proactive steps to filter out some higher-risk individuals:

➤ Deputize the entire student body to become the eyes-and-ears safety net for the school. To do so, they must come to understand that "telling is not tattling." They need to understand that anyone whom they bring to the attention of the right people will get much-needed help and support. So we need to deputize our young people and instill in them the understanding that tattling isn't telling, it's providing compassionate help.

➤ A truly anonymous text and phone hotline should be established to alert school officials to male students causing concern among their peers.

➤ Qualified professionals should react to those contacts and investigate to see how many factors above are present and make contact with the student in the most nurturing and supportive way possible. Once most individuals get past their crisis point, they seldom return to that low point.

➤ Also intervene with family to make efforts to resolve dysfunction in the home and, above all else, lock up or remove the guns from the home. Alert friends and family to do the same.

Using the above criteria, the challenge can become manageable.

With just the insights I've discussed here, consider a school with 800 students.

Roughly half are girls, so the group of concern is immediately cut to 400.

Ages between sixteen and nineteen cuts it to roughly 250–280.

Now apply the other identifiers and you can eliminate the boys on sports teams, debate team, choir, and other engaging activities, because they are not marginalized. The high-risk individuals have *observable* psychological problems. Now you are down to a small number of those who need monitoring.

Remember these people also tell someone who can be sensitized to come forward.

We also know the shooters tend to strike on the twentieth of the month, with January being the most frequent month.

Perhaps the most important element that we need is a massive public push/educational program about gun lockup and storage at home. I'm a gun owner and I don't know a single gun owner who has a problem with this.

All of these steps are achievable, affordable, commonsensical, and noncontroversial. The fact that we haven't undertaken such a plan with any sort of national urgency is just a painful, brutal reminder that the desire to win an argument is preventing us from doing all we can be doing to solve a problem. This is a mandate.

Solving a Problem Means Picking Your Battles

There's an old saying that to have a happy marriage, you only have to give your wife one thing: her way. That's funny, and it may even have some truth to it, but if I had to tell you the key reason I've stayed married for forty-seven years, it's that I picked my battles.

And guess what? You don't have to pick every one. This isn't just true for marriage. It's true for all of us, in every situation—from the ridiculous to the deadly serious.

You do not need to react every time somebody says something that goes in your ear sideways. When I say pick your battles, that means:

- Pick which issues you think need to be confronted and leave the others alone
- Pick your time
- Pick your place
- Pick your rules or methods of engagement
- Most importantly, pick your outcome criteria

You don't have to fight the battle just because somebody throws a hoe handle down and wants to fight with you. In fact, I would argue that those are the worst battles to fight because you're allowing someone else to pick the time and the place, and, as far as you know, their only criterion for a successful outcome is that you rose to the bait. You can wait until you have your thoughts together. You may even want to gather some evidence or make some notes.

Easier said than done, I know. It's tough to learn to let something roll off your back. But it's important.

Awhile back, on *Dr. Phil*, I had an opportunity to speak with a mother from Detroit who was terrified for the safety of her two sons—Tywonn and Naybon. Both sons were college students. Tywonn was studying criminal justice. Naybon was in law school.

Around midnight one night, the boys headed out to get food, and police officers began tailing their car. When they pulled into the restaurant, the officers followed them in and asked to see their identification.

Tywonn and Naybon asked what they had done wrong. Naybon pointed out that he was a law student, and he knew his rights.

This infuriated the police officers, who reached out to grab one of the brothers—at which point the other knocked away his hand.[3]

At that point, it became a full-on fistfight—and to make things even more dangerous, Tywonn and Naybon were winning. Mom came to talk to me looking for help in providing some real-world guidance to her sons, who had both agreed to come with her. When I tell you these were two of the nicest, well-raised young men, I mean it. Please go to my YouTube channel and search their names—their story will pop right up—and judge for yourself. Any parent, Black or white, single or married, would be proud to claim these two fine young men.

Their story was consistent but clearly not coached or rehearsed. They both maintained that the minute the police officers started throwing punches at them, they were no longer police officers.[4]

I could not have disagreed more. "Sorry, boys, you are wrong." (And that's a good way to be "dead wrong"!) I told them that you can get their name, you can get their badge number, you can ask for the security footage—but you do not throw a punch. You may think you're winning a fight, but that's not a fight you're ever going to win. Ever. So when "a badge" tells you to do something, whether you like it or not, the *safest* thing to do is comply in the moment. Do not give a person who has a badge and a gun a reason to use either on you. Decide what you are going to do in that circumstance before you are in it.

- ➤ They have governmental authority, you do not.
- ➤ They have a badge, you do not.
- ➤ They have Mace, a billy club, a Taser, and handcuffs. You do not.

➤ They have a radio to call twenty more who are equipped the same way. You do not.

➤ They have a gun, a lethal weapon. You do not.

If Vegas was handicapping this fight, at this time, on this battle-field, I think even Beavis and Butthead could pick the winner!

Now, the emotional argument is so easy that I can make your *emotional* argument better than you:

➤ But we weren't doing anything wrong.

➤ We have rights.

➤ They were outside the scope of their employment, job description, and authority.

➤ They were just assaulting us like a mugger.

➤ YOU, Dr. Phil, say, "Don't reward bad behavior." If we let them get away with this, aren't we doing just that?

➤ If we don't stand up for ourselves like men, who will?

I agree with every point I just listed. You do have rights, they were outside the scope, you did get assaulted, you would be reward-ing bad behavior if you let them get away with it, and you would be betraying yourselves if you didn't fight back. (Notice I gave a legiti-mate version of their argument. I did not mock it or make fun of it. It was important to me that they understood that I heard them, but still disagreed.)

My two key points—and they are *huge* ones—are simply time and place. Don't give your power away. Do not let them pick the time and place. You pick it. I have one and only one measure of success: get you home *alive.* If you get back to your mother, *alive,* that is a win, a big win. You can say, "Setting the bar pretty low there, aren't you, Dr. Phil?" The answer would be yes *if* the story ended there. But on my timeline, it is just beginning. Because *now YOU* are in control and you are picking the time, the place, the weapons, the outcome measures. Their advantages are *gone.* They are not going to shoot, tase, club, or kill you in a courtroom. They are going to get called out, humiliated, and then write you a big check.

Especially when it comes to dealing with police who are mistreating you, your choice couldn't be simpler: there is a bag in your future. Fight on their terms and it could be a body bag. Fight on your terms and it could be a money bag. And you have made a record that could have a profound impact on whether they keep that badge (and if so, *how* they use it with the next two young men they encounter).

If you don't believe me, if you believe all the hateful hype in some of the print press or electronic media, you will be missing some important facts.

In the interest of full transparency, and I said as much to Ty and Naybon, I am an outspoken supporter of law enforcement. The vast majority of the approximately 800,000 men and women who wear that badge in America every day to maintain order and keep the rest of us safe.

I absolutely abhor the "badge-heavy" bullies who abuse their power and victimize the public, disproportionately minorities, especially young Black men.

But this is key: many of the abusers are held accountable *when you pick the right battlefield.* In the decade between 2012 and 2022, twenty-five of the largest police and sheriff's departments in America paid a whopping $3.2 billion to resolve claims of misconduct.[5] That massive amount of money says a lot of things. It says that police departments are getting called out for misconduct—and paying for it. It says those funds would probably be better spent on screening and training that prevents the misconduct in the first place. But for the purposes of our story here, the message is very clear: if you are a victim of misconduct, stay calm, *stay alive,* and then fight the battle on your terms.

Luckily, the two brothers didn't get killed. But they were arrested for assault on a police officer.

And then they fought the battle they wanted to fight. They got the footage. They got their story on TV. The prosecutor dropped the charges. And the brothers won a settlement.

You can solve a lot more things if you react to fewer of them. Pick your battles and everything associated with fighting one.

POLL RESPONSE

If you're being totally honest with yourself, when you are in conflict with someone you care about, how often are you focused on being right/winning the argument, rather than solving the problem?

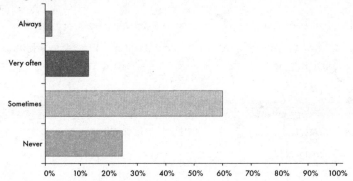

I don't often begin a survey question with a qualifier like "If you're being totally honest with yourself," but in this case it's warranted—because your knee-jerk reaction might be different from your honest, thoughtful, self-assessment. On this one, I'm speaking from experience!

PRINCIPLE #3

Do Not Reward Bad Behavior or Support Conduct You Do Not Value

---

POLL QUESTION

Do you ever give a child a treat to stop them from crying, complaining, or interrupting; or to a pet to stop them from whining or scratching?

- ☐ Always
- ☐ Very often
- ☐ Sometimes
- ☐ Never

Several years ago, I did an episode of *Dr. Phil* on autism or autism spectrum disorder.

Now, autism is a developing field of study, and it can be a controversial and politically charged issue within the medical, psychiatric, and psychological professions. There are different groups supporting different philosophies as to diagnostic criteria, classifications, and treatment protocols.

After the show, one group sent me a thoughtful letter, explaining where they thought I hadn't fully covered something they felt was important.

So I wrote them back and said, "Hey, good point. We'll do another show on this soon. I'd love to have you on and give you an opportunity to talk about that in a more fulsome manner. Thanks for contributing; the more information we can get out there the better."

There was another group, who saw things somewhat differently than the one who wrote in, who also had an issue, and they took a different approach. They didn't write me a letter or contact my staff. They instead ran to the media, tried to turn it into a media event, attempted to stir up turmoil, and used that to try to elevate their own profile, if they even had one.

In this case, my staff asked, "Should we have them on too?"

I said, "Never in a million years."

You don't reward bad behavior. I would have been willing to give both sides a chance to educate the public. Clearly that was not their agenda.

It seems obvious, not rewarding bad behavior. But in life and society, we reward bad behavior *all the time*.

When a child is having a tantrum, you don't give them a cookie to quiet them down.

That's because behavior is influenced by its consequences, and sometimes we unintentionally reinforce bad behavior. The first time your dog scratches on the cabinet where you keep the treats, you think it's cute, so you give him a treat. But now he knows that if he scratches on the cabinet, he gets a treat. Congratulations, you've unintentionally provided positive reinforcement for a behavior that will require you to repaint your cabinet every year.

Again, we reward bad behavior all the time. In elementary schools, I've seen children who were sent to the office to be punished allowed to

> **It seems obvious, not rewarding bad behavior. But in life and society, we reward bad behavior *all the time*.**

sit and watch cartoons on an iPad. I've seen football coaches give more playing time to players who play dirty. Those are individual examples, but we also reward bad behavior on a societal scale. We plow more money into schools that are failing and continue to fund programs that don't get results. We give CEOs and coaches who get fired massive paydays, we put bad cops back on the streets—the list goes on and on.

To me, one of the most important examples of rewarding bad behavior today is in the area of addiction and an approach called "harm reduction."

When someone close to you is in crisis or is addicted to drugs and you give them money or a place to stay, you're rewarding bad behavior.

You may tell yourself, "I give her money because I want her to be safe." But actually, you're giving her money so *you* feel better. To reduce your own anxiety—you're actually putting your own needs ahead of hers.

On a larger scale, that's basically the idea behind the school of thought known as "harm reduction."

Harm reduction policies and approaches typically claim to attempt to minimize the negative health, social, and legal impacts associated with drug use, drug policies, and drug laws.[1] To be sure, there's a lot of harm to reduce. Overdose deaths in this country are going through the roof. Since 1999, the number has quintupled, and it is still rising.

In 2022, the last year for which we have records, overdose deaths in this country topped 105,000, according to the National Institutes of Health (NIH).[2] That's over three hundred people a day, the equivalent of a jumbo jet going down every day. And you'd better bet if a plane was crashing every day, we'd be doing everything we could to get a handle on the airline industry.

The tragic toll of these overdoses has led to the spread of several different kinds of harm reduction approaches across the country. For example, these programs might provide drug users with a safe place to use drugs, or clean needles so users who inject drugs are less likely to get HIV or other infections, or testing to make sure the drugs they're using aren't laced with fentanyl, or the facilities will have on hand a drug called Narcan, which can save the life of someone who has overdosed.

Fans of harm reduction will say that they're being pragmatic, that they're working within the reality that there will always be addicts. They're not trying to create a drug-free society; they argue that drugs and addiction are inevitable. The goal is to reduce the number of overdose deaths, and by that measure, these programs are effective.

To me, supporting harm reduction that reduces overdose deaths is like playing a game that a child makes up. They make the rules, they define victory, and they always win. Reducing overdose deaths has nothing to say about the other costs of addiction. What about the ongoing trauma an addict causes their family? What about the chances that someone who is high on drugs gets in their car and causes a terrible accident?

As the biomedical ethicist Nicholas King writes, "If we are to be truly utilitarian about our assessment of these programs, it is worth asking whether, on balance, the harm reduced by preventing an overdose death actually outweighs the harms of continuing to use illegal drugs, living with an addiction, and causing continued suffering to those who are addicted and their families and caregivers."[3]

In that sense, harm reduction is enabling harmful behavior. In fact, while safe injection sites offer a safer way to use illegal, deadly, substances, in my view they do not offer near enough opportunity to seek freedom from those substances. They give lip service to it, they say they have counselors available, but in practice the focus is too much on safe injection and not enough on overcoming the disease.

One study found that fewer than 7 percent of users of safe injection sites accept referrals to any kind of addiction treatment.[4] And why would they? There's no incentive to get off drugs if you're being provided with a warm, safe place to do them. That is the definition of rewarding bad behavior. And when we reward bad behavior, other people get hurt. Because safe injection sites reduce only one kind of "harm." They don't focus on restoring the person to wholeness or wellness—physically, mentally, spiritually, or socially.[5]

Unlike integrated addiction programs, there is not near enough, if any, work done to help the person address their addiction, restore the person to health, help them take responsibility or make amends, or help them make choices that will help their overall well-being.

When we support programs like this, we're not alleviating harm; we're cooperating in harm. These programs just make it easier for addicts to get deeper into the addiction. They erode their organ function further. The drugs hijack their pleasure center even more, while the addict deepens the habitual nature of their conduct.

At some point they need to quit. It doesn't get easier the longer they practice the bad habit.

We're condoning drug abuse, which impedes the ability of the human person to think well and act responsibly. We're actively encouraging a habit that destroys bodies, minds, and lives, and which harms families and communities.

We miss an opportunity to free people from drug abuse and addiction because supervised injecting rooms, in order to attract clients, avoid any strong message about abstinence and rehabilitation.

We might even be *encouraging* drug abuse by offering a secure venue for the practice.

There's also the risk that we're encouraging drug trafficking by giving dealers and users a law-enforcement-free location for their trade.

Some studies even show that harm reduction destabilizes communities by reducing property values of the surrounding homes and businesses.

And we take a step toward decriminalizing and normalizing "hard" drugs.

Harm reduction sees no overdoses as 100 percent success. And if that's your measure of success—if that's your outcome criterion—you get an A-plus. But to me, that's just surrendering to the disease. You're on one end of the rope, the disease is on the other, and harm reduction is us just dropping the rope and saying, "We're just going to manage the disease."

The goal should be to get people off the drugs. Period.

That's just one example, and there are countless others. Try to think of some other places where you see individuals or society rewarding—or even subsidizing—bad behavior. That way you can steer clear of harmful incentive structures in your own life and help our country get back to encouraging healthy behavior in us all.

POLL RESPONSE

Do you ever give a child a treat to stop them from crying, complaining, or interrupting; or to a pet to stop them from whining or scratching?

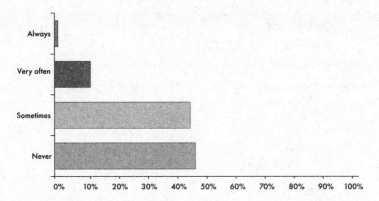

Measure All Actions Based on Results and All Thoughts Based on Rationality

---

POLL QUESTIONS

How frequently do you question or measure whether your behavior patterns, projects, and pursuits in life are working or not? (This is not based on your opinion or perception, but on measurable outcomes.)

☐ Always
☐ Very often
☐ Sometimes
☐ Never

What proportion of your decisions would you say you make based on emotional reactions (versus logical or rational analysis)?

☐ All of them
☐ Most of them
☐ A handful of them
☐ None of them

If you've spent any time listening to me, there's one question you've heard more than any other.

Say it with me: "How's that working for you?"

It's not a catchphrase. I mean it sincerely.

Every action you take, every decision you make, should be based on results.

If it ain't working out, it ain't working.

Growing up, I had a paper route in the morning and afternoons. That means I was up at four o'clock in the morning on school days. And I'd go throw my paper route. We lived in Oklahoma City at the time, and one night it was sleeting. I mean cold, freezing rain, wind; everything was moving horizontally. It was just not fit for man nor beast outside.

I was putting my coat on, getting ready to head out, and my mother said, "Where are you going?" I said, "I'm going to collect for the paper." And she said, "Not tonight you're not. Are you crazy?" I said, "No, I'm not. Everybody's home tonight."

For me, this was a target-rich environment. Usually when you went to collect for the paper, you had to go back time and time again, because people weren't home. And when they were home, they'd get a bit frustrated with you for asking for your $1.15, which was the monthly cost for the *Daily Oklahoman* at the time. By the way, there were no plastic bags, so when it rained you had to roll the newspaper in wax paper to protect it, to keep it from getting soggy. But when I knocked on doors in that storm, all my customers were home. Seeing me, dripping wet and freezing cold, they felt grateful (and probably a little sympathetic) for what I was doing to get them their papers.

And so on that night I said, "I'm collecting for the paper for this month and the next two months." A few of them said, "Oh, I didn't know you did that." I replied, "Well, it's just to be convenient for you."

So I had my customers set up to pay three months at a time—four times a year—rather than twelve. Going out on one rough night got me paid and saved me a lot of time and energy.

Result: a lesson well learned and never forgotten.

I've been results-oriented as long as I can remember. When you grow up poor you become *very* results oriented. You can't go to the grocery store with "good intentions." You can't tell the clerk, "*I intended to work today.* I don't have any money but since I *intended* to work today, is that good enough to get these groceries?"

I was poor enough that I knew *working* today was not even good enough. I had to also *get paid today* or I would not eat. That's what I mean when I say that you learn to be very *results-oriented.* And I learned it from a very young age. There was no credit, no good intention, no "somebody else should fix this for me." There was only "CIF"—cash in fist!

My focus on results is why, early in my career, I consciously decided to take a different approach to helping people struggling with psychological issues. Some had personal issues, some had relationship issues, while others had social issues or addiction issues. It seemed the challenges were endless.

Some therapists are comfortable and effective in a nondirectional or reflective model. The patient or client might say something like "My marriage isn't working, and my husband yells at me" and the therapist would respond, "How does that make you feel?"

They would do that for six months, and never once would the therapist ask their patient to do anything direct. For some it is a very effective therapeutic model that leads to self-discovery.

I've never been that way.

I've always been very action-oriented and directive—within the context of an evidence-based therapeutic model.

My colleagues, early on in my practice, would half-jokingly say, "You fix these people in three days, you're going to run out of patients, and you're going to run out of money."

That's not what happened.

The truth was I had a long waiting list because people wanted answers; they wanted direction they could work hard to implement.

These were people who didn't just want to talk about changes; they wanted to make changes and learn and grow experientially.

This approach wasn't for everyone. I'm not even saying it was better. But it was different, and it certainly worked for me and for most of the people I worked with.

The therapists and the patients who were drawn to that approach believed in self-direction and self-determination. They wanted to see results.

They wanted to see evidence rather than join an ideology.

They were asking the question we need to ask in so many areas: "Is what we're doing working?"

Is it worth the time?

Is it worth the attention?

Is it worth the money?

Think about these questions across our country today.

What have we "paid" to fight climate change and what are we getting?

What have tax cuts cost us, and what are they doing for the economy?

What are we doing to fight homelessness, and is it working?

The same goes for drugs (as we just discussed) and crime, and immigration, and gun violence. I don't want to hear about the process. I don't want to hear about the intention. Show me the results. And if you can't show me results, show me a new plan.

One of the clearest examples of paying for intention, despite truly horrendous, damaging results, is in education.

We live in a country where 130 million adults can't read a simple story. Nineteen percent of high school graduates can't read. This isn't just their problem, it's all of ours. More than 40 percent of "low-literate" adults live in poverty, compared to only 5 percent of people at the highest literacy.[1] And it's a cycle—nearly a quarter of unemployed people in America are low-literate. They can't find work because they can't read, which leads to poverty. They are unable to read to their children, and their children are more likely to end up in poverty.

Early in 2023, the Illinois State Board of Education posted the Illinois Schools 2022 Report Card on their website.[2] It's a massive spreadsheet full of data—everything from teacher salaries to teacher experience, to class size, to absentee rates, to incidents of violence in schools, to the number of students who are "on track" and the number of students who take Advanced Placement classes.

I'll give the Illinois State Board of Education credit on this point: they certainly ain't trying to hide anything.

Every bit of information they have, they've put it out there. *Dragnet*-style: just the facts. But that's where the good news ends, because an organization called Wirepoints, which aims "to be a place for independent thinkers who challenge orthodoxy with facts," started digging into the data.

Wirepoints says that its mission is "relentlessly questioning current assumptions, and changing accordingly when they prove wrong. We're not here to make any friends on the left or the right. We call things as we see them."[3] My kind of organization.

Well, here's what the crew from Wirepoints noticed when they dug into the data. In fifty-three Illinois schools, not a single student could do math at grade level. Fifty-three schools, not one student. In reading, there were thirty schools where not a single student could read at grade level. Thirty schools, not one student.

By the way, there are another 622 schools where less than 10 percent of the children can read at grade level. And another 930 schools—more than a quarter of all schools in the state—where less than 10 percent of children can do math at grade level.

It's not just Illinois. In Baltimore, twenty-three schools have zero students proficient in math.[4]

How is this possible? What is the cause?

It's not necessarily what you'd think.

You can't pin this on the pandemic. Wirepoints looked at the example of one school, called Spry, where not a single student is at grade level in reading or math. Before the pandemic, only two students could read at grade level, and zero were proficient in math. Now, this school could argue that the pandemic "made things worse"—and I suppose going from two students who can read to zero students who can read is "worse." But c'mon—this school hadn't lifted any children off the floor, and, as I've said before, you can't fall off the floor.

You can't pin this on lack of money. Before the pandemic, spending at that one school was nearly $20,000 per student. Then, with city and federal funding, it went up to more than $35,000 per student. That's more than the average private school in Illinois.

Let me repeat that: the state of Illinois was paying more than it would cost to send a child to private school to send them to public school, where they weren't learning to read.

We're not seeing stories like this everywhere, thank God. But we are seeing examples like this in too many places, and not just inner cities. The National Assessment of Educational Progress says 32 percent of fourth graders and 24 percent of eighth graders can't read beyond even the most basic level.

I'm sure the *intent* of the board of education is to teach children. I'm sure that the *intent* of the teachers is to teach children. But the result is that students aren't getting taught. So we need to ask, what's going to get us a better result?

It's going to involve things like year-round school, training and supporting teachers to help them to be more effective, and working extensively with parents to make sure they can reinforce what's being taught in the classroom. It's also going to require that we recognize that we don't have time for blue-ribbon panels or special commissions. You can't take it under advisement; the situation is urgent.

Every day you wait, students fall further behind.

So we're measuring actions based on results.

And the best way to get the results you want is to make sure that you're building on a foundation of rational thought.

It's amazing how often I talk to someone who's frustrated about an outcome in their life that's the result of an irrational thought or expectation at the front end.

One of my favorite and most extreme examples of this comes from Richard Feynman, who was a theoretical physicist who won the Nobel Prize. He was a big brain, and physicists will tell you that his contributions to the field were huge. They'll tell you a lot more than that, but it's all beyond my understanding. In 1964 he gave a lecture he called "Seeking New Laws."[5] It's mostly heavy physics stuff. But when it came to solving physics problems, he offered an approach that applies to so much more. He said, "We are trying to prove ourselves wrong as quickly as possible, because only in that way can we find progress."

Feynman's expertise was physics, but he also knew a lot about human nature. A few years later, in 1974, he gave the commencement speech at the California Institute of Technology.[6] It is the kind of speech that would absolutely get someone cancelled today. (He starts the speech by describing his inability to figure out the best pickup line to use on a woman he meets in a hot tub. You see, back then consenting adults could actually banter back and forth. It was called "flirting," and it was quite popular.) But then he turns his attention to all the things we believe because we think they're somewhat scientific, but they're not. We think they're based on evidence, but they're not.

In the speech, he uses the example of the "cargo cults." During World War II, lots of islands in the South Pacific saw American planes and American troops for the first time.[7] Residents saw these planes land and unload all sorts of things that seemed almost magical. Jeeps and new types of food, and lights.

So, what happened? Feynman describes a scene where, years later, in some places, the people built imitations of runways, with fires alongside them, and a little hut for a man to sit in, with two wooden pieces on his head made to look like headphones, and sticks of bamboo made to look like antennas. And then they waited for the planes to start landing.

But no airplanes landed.

What went wrong?

Everything looked the way it looked when airplanes landed the first time. That's what Feynman called "cargo cult science." It looks scientific, but it isn't. It looks rational—"if I re-create the conditions where planes landed the first time, they'll land again." Of course, we immediately see that it's not rational at all. It's easier to see irrational thought when we're looking at someone else; it's harder when we're looking at ourselves.

In fact, Feynman makes that point in his speech. We teach people lots of things, but the one thing we don't teach them is how *to not fool themselves*. Because once you believe something to be true, you start to either ignore or fudge inconvenient facts that don't align with that belief. So, as he sent these idealistic young graduates into the world, he reminded them: "The first principle is that you must not fool yourself—and you are the easiest person to fool."

You may wonder why that is. Why are you so easy to fool?

It's quite simple.

In order to get through life, it is pretty much a necessity that we believe ourselves. We trust that when we tell ourselves something, it is true. It has to work that way or else we would never be able to even move about in the world.

Think about it: If you believe the next step you take will fall on solid, safe ground, you will willingly take that next step. If, on the other hand, you believe the next step you take will be into thin air and you will fall ten stories and die, you will fight with every ounce of strength you have to keep from taking that next step.

I know it's a simple example (although it's a real one—there are actual studies showing that babies won't crawl onto a glass ledge), but think about how that translates into other things you believe and act on in your life.

Whatever you're telling yourself about your abilities, other people's integrity, someone's representations to you about the safety of an investment, someone's intentions with your children, the truthfulness of an ideology—you are likely to believe. How could you not? Otherwise you'd be paralyzed by self-doubt, unable to make even the simplest decisions.

What you tell yourself about so many different things can be absolutely outcome-determinative in your life.

You have good intentions.

You mean to tell yourself the truth.

You believe wholeheartedly you're dealing in facts.

But what if in reality you're not?

The "what if" game involves playing out any given scenario all the way to the end, step by step. You ask yourself "what if" about each possible outcome or result. This is one place where playing the "what if?" game can actually be very healthy and helpful. Ask yourself how often you really put those things that you're accepting as "factual" to the test.

Are you checking things out as much as you really should? And, associated with that, what are the stakes?

Sometimes what you tell yourself can be no big deal. If, for example, you're talking to yourself about a movie or restaurant, the worst outcome is that you end up with a bad meal or waste a couple of hours at a movie you didn't really enjoy. But then again, it can be something deeply profound. Like whether to believe what you are telling *yourself* about your child's story about where they have been or what happened to them. Or what your government is telling you about what they are doing or what you should do.

The only way to know for sure is to test your thoughts.

I want to underline the distinction I am making here. I am not focusing on evaluating the rationality of what you are being told, although that is of course always good to do.

I'm focusing on what you *say to yourself* about what is being said to you.

It is so important that you actively listen to yourself with an evaluative mindset, not be on "automatic pilot," and actively test the rationality of your thoughts. If you distort your perception, silence that little voice that's whispering warnings, or lie to yourself—even by omission—you can defeat yourself in life.

If we want to build a stronger America, we have to build it on a foundation of rational thought.

There are several principles that underlie rational thought, and the first and most fundamental is that the simplest explanation is often the correct one. This principle has been around in one form or another since ancient times, and today goes by such names as the Principle of Parsimony or Occam's razor. It boils down to this: when you're dealing with competing hypotheses or explanations, you should lean toward the one that requires fewer variables and assumptions. During my training, one of my professors often reminded us, "If you hear hoofbeats, think horses, not zebras."

If you see an unusual light in the sky, it could be an alien spacecraft from millions of light-years away signaling the beginning of an invasion, *orrrrrr* it could be a weather balloon.

> **If you distort your perception, silence that little voice that's whispering warnings, or lie to yourself—even by omission—you can defeat yourself in life.**

A mysterious click on your phone while you're talking could mean it is bugged, *orrrrr* it could be static because you are in a lousy reception area.

Black SUVs might be following you, *orrrr* half the cars in that part of town could be black SUVs.

We could have gotten the definition of sex wrong for thousands of years, despite all chromosomal evidence to the contrary . . . *orrrr* it could be that a group with a self-referential agenda is trying to validate how they see themselves, and who have changed their own definitions of gender and sex over the last several years.

You can argue about each of these, and Lord knows people do.

Some things just are what they are, and some things just are not. And if you need to determine if you're thinking rationally beyond Occam's razor, I would advise you to simply check your thoughts against these four criteria.

Isolate a given thought, something you are telling yourself, and test it by asking *and answering* four questions about that thought. And guess what, number one is what I have just been writing about:

1. Is it based on empirical, verifiable fact or criteria?
2. Is this in my best interest?
3. Does it get me what I want?
4. Does it protect and prolong my life?

You quickly see how the cargo cult thoughts and the behaviors they led to fail on every count.

It looked like it might be based on empirical facts or criteria, but it clearly wasn't. Having those uninformed thoughts and expending the energy to dig up the jungle to build an imitation of a runway that no plane was ever going to land on was not in anyone's best interest.

It didn't get the people who believed in it what they wanted.

It didn't offer any protection or improvement to their lives.

It was based on an unchallenged and faulty belief about cause and effect.

What does this sort of backward thinking have to do with us? Everything.

I'm about to tell you a factually verified story that *involves* COVID, but it is not really *about* COVID. It's a story you probably haven't heard. It really has little to do with the disease at all (which you're probably tired of hearing about) and a whole lot to do with the people who recklessly hijacked your life.

As you read through this brief overview, let's remember two relevant concepts:

1. The Hippocratic Oath, which I mentioned earlier in relation to doctors providing gender transition care: "First, do no harm." A twenty-first-century adaptation of a much more elaborate oath of medical ethics found in ancient Greek medical texts. Pretty simple, right? "Doctor, whatever you do, *first do no harm.*"

2. Fiduciary duty: When an individual, agency, or organization has a duty to put your interest ahead of their own. In his article "The Fiduciary Obligations of Public Officials," Vincent R. Johnson states clearly, "Regardless of whether specific rules of government ethics have been adopted, public officials have a broad fiduciary duty to carry out their responsibilities in a manner that is faithful to the public trust that has been reposed in them."

With those two concepts in mind, this becomes a story not about helping you and your family, but of actual harm, power, control, lost perspective, and whether our government officials' response to the disease *was rational.*

I'm obviously not going to hide the ball or tease the ending—it demonstrably was not.

So let's start from the beginning. Actually, let's start before the beginning.

Between 2009 and 2021, all *prepandemic years*, the share of American high school students who said they felt "persistent feelings of sadness or hopelessness" rose from 26 percent to 44 percent, according to a study by the Centers for Disease Control and Prevention (CDC). That is a 59 percent increase! And experience tells us it is very likely *under*reported.

This is the highest level of teenage sadness ever recorded.[8] For everyone involved with this population, understanding and confronting this phenomenon had to be job number one.

In 2017, 13 percent of teenagers between the ages of twelve and seventeen (that's roughly 3.2 million young people) said they had experienced at least one major depressive episode in the past year, up from 8 percent (2 million) in 2007. That's 1.2 million more depressive episodes in 2017 than in 2007.

The total number of teenagers who recently experienced depression increased 59 percent between 2007 and 2017—with the faster growth among teen girls.[9] A study by the CDC found that between 2011 and 2021, the number of teen girls who reported experiencing sadness and hopelessness went from 36 percent to 59 percent. This all had to be center screen on everyone's "Red Alert Radar." This is an epidemic-level, nationwide trend that is costing lives, diminishing quality of life, and showing no signs of letting up or improving.

It is seriously disrupting learning and thereby undercutting preparation for the next level of life. Put simply, it is putting an entire generation at risk. It calls for drastic measures. This is exactly why we devote billions of dollars to agencies such as the Department of Education and the CDC.

So, our school-age children are suffering, which begs the question, why?

Clearly there has to be more than one reason, although we know there's at least one strong correlation between how much they're suffering and how much they're using social media.

But there are a lot of reasons for this that go beyond social media and young people getting tunnel vision by looking down at their phones instead of up at the world.

Whatever the case, the point is that we knew that this trend was there and has, in fact, been accelerating for over ten years.

It was no secret to our educators, mental health professionals, and governmental agencies that our school-age children were in a chronic and deepening crisis. It is also known that social interaction with peers, participation in academic and classroom activities, extracurricular activities, the satisfaction of gaining knowledge through academic achievement, to physical activity (everything from a walk around the neighborhood to team sports)—all of these are critical to fighting off loneliness, depression, and anxiety.

Those developmental activities are extremely important building blocks in the growth of children mentally, emotionally, and socially. It is also no secret that isolation is the antithesis of mental health.

So, in summary, here is what was known by decision makers 100 percent for sure: we have a delicate and vulnerable generation of students, suffering at historically high levels (with children from lower socioeconomic and minority backgrounds suffering the worst), in desperate need of greater real-world activity and social interaction.

And then COVID comes along.

And what do our *fiduciaries* do?

Starting in March 2020, they shut down the schools. They sent the kids home—where they have *nothing but* screens and social media and less physical activity, a known contributor to the crisis.

I understand, thinking back to that March, that there was a ton of fear and uncertainty. So I had no problem with the powers that be taking a pause for a week and saying, "Okay, all hands on deck. Let's figure this out." It's not going to ruin anybody's life to call timeout for a week, even two, but let's remember we have to weigh the impact of this virus against the impact of isolating a highly vulnerable, already hurting generation of students.

But our leaders did not do that. They did not weigh the relative threat of one against the other. They discovered that they had the power to shut down the world (and the schools with it)—and they did this not for two weeks but for two years!

And they didn't do it to save the lives of children who were vulnerable to some dread disease for whom going to school would be certain death. Long after these decision makers knew that the disease didn't present a particular risk to young people, they persisted in keeping the schools closed. And the vast majority of those children will be paying the price for that reckless, politicized decision-making for decades to come.

I'm sorry, but there's just no excuse for that. There is no justification, there is no equivocation, there is no "we did the best we could with what we knew at the time" argument. No, you didn't.

It was just such nonsense, when there were such sensible solutions available.

Have class outside, wherever and whenever that was possible.

If teachers were at particular risk, let them teach the virtual classes to kids who might also have been out sick.

But instead, what did we do?

We take children who were already struggling with anxiety, depression, and loneliness—and put them into isolation! Four walls and a screen. More time for social media. Less mandatory exercise. More of the things that were hurting them, and less of what was helping them.

Lassie could figure this one out. You can't tell me the Department of Education, CDC, state school boards, teachers' unions, everyone charged with safeguarding our young people's mental and physical health could not connect these dots.

Again, we know that for children's healthy growth and development, they need interaction; they need social experiences; they need to be with their peers and doing in-classroom learning—with less time on screens and social media.

We know this is particularly important for children who are minorities or from lower socioeconomic backgrounds—because in many cases they are in environments where there may only be one parent, or both parents are working, or they might have poor internet connections. Their chance to keep up or make progress under remote learning is so slim you're just throwing them under the bus—assuming the bus was running at all, which it wasn't.

This deprived them of something else they were getting from school: food, shelter, safety.

These kids were already swinging on a frayed safety net, and we just put a knife to it.

Many of these children were depending on two meals a day from the schools, and they shut those schools down.

Now some heroic school bus drivers drove their routes, not picking up kids but handing out meals. And some schools said, "Well, we made the meals available at the community center." But in a lot of cases, kids went without.

And, by the way, if they could go to a community center to have two meals, why couldn't they go to a classroom and have classes? That made about as much sense as shutting down churches but leaving open pornography stores and marijuana dispensaries!

Meanwhile, a bad response to one risk only heightened another: the referrals for sexual molestation and physical abuse dropped as much as 65 percent during the lockdown. And trust me, that's not because the abuse and molestation weren't happening. It was because "mandated reporters"—the teachers, coaches, counselors, administrators, and other state employees who are contractually obligated to report suspicions of abuse—did not have eyes on these students to report those red-flag warnings.

Think of the daily hell of being locked in with your abuser! That was the reality for a lot of these children. They were fed to the wolves. Who was thinking for the people making these decisions?

And that doesn't even begin to touch what hell this was on parents, mostly moms, and especially the moms who had to work and had no way to balance caregiving and work.[10]

So, what kept our children out of school?

It certainly did not take two years to figure out that the risk to children's lives from the virus were not anywhere near the levels of risk to their lives from depression and isolation, or that measures could be taken to protect the teachers. First-line responders, nurses, paramedics, EMTs, doctors, and hospital personnel found a way and kept the system working. Essential workers in many other industries such as grocery stores found a way, but not our schools, where we knew the children were already suffering mentally and emotionally and prolonged shutdowns would be highly exacerbating?

These agencies blew it. They blew it big-time. It's astounding that they have budgets and bureaucracies that grow every year, theoretically "building capacity" to take on big challenges. Then, when it's finally their time to step up and manage the kind of crisis they exist to be ready for, they fumble so badly that a generation may well be damaged irreparably. Shame on them.

So, again, why? Why did they not do their jobs? They can read, and oftentimes the research was their own! They were telling themselves and all of us that these children were in crisis. So, who kept the kids out of the schools and why?

Not the teachers—they were amazing. They learned how to teach on Zoom, they checked in on their kids, they did the best they could.

And they paid a price—by one measure, a quarter of them wanted to leave their jobs by the end of that first pandemic year.[11]

The problem was not with the teachers; the problem was with the teachers' *unions*. It became not a scientific issue, or a public health issue, or an epidemiological issue—it became a political issue, and the schools opened in inverse proportionality to the strength of the teachers' unions in control in a given region. The stronger the union, the slower the schools were to open.[12]

A group of powerful people basically put their members on a semi-strike and did lifelong damage to millions of students. Speaking of life and millions, pediatric epidemiologist Dr. Dimitri Christakis is the director of the Center for Child Health, Behavior and Development at Seattle Children's Research Institute. He has authored a pediatrics textbook as well as more than 170 original research articles. He has created models that quantify and predict the health impact of this overextended quarantine. The models predict that the toll on these innocent children will be as many as 15 to 17 million years of life lost.[13] That's a result of the mental and emotional damage they've suffered, the lower educational attainment they'll achieve, and the different career paths that spring from all of that. Millions of years of life lost and diminished. What a tragedy. What an unnecessary tragedy.

As I have said, I always focus on why people do what they do, and don't do what they don't do. You really have to ask yourself what motivated the forces at play here. It sure wasn't the Hippocratic Oath and they sure weren't acting as fiduciaries.

The only answers left: too much power and too little perspective.

Think of the power that a couple of small groups wielded at that moment in history. Literally a handful of people at a conference table could sit down and say: "We have the power to shut down this entire country. We can sit here and shut down America."

And then they do it, and all of a sudden, the entire world comes to a halt, and there's no smog over LA, and animals start coming out of hiding—and there's some belief that you're saving mankind.

And that's where the loss of perspective comes in—because the CDC, based on results, never really considered the lives that would be lost and the suffering that would take place *because* of the lockdown, the small businesses and the dreams they represented wiped off the map in an instant. Sadly, some surveys reported that 60 percent of small businesses that had to close due to the COVID shutdown never reopened regardless of how long they had been in business.[14] In some cases, generations of work were wiped away by an unscientific bureaucratic decision. The same way the teachers' unions didn't consider how much they'd be hurting students and teachers. The response was, in a word, irrational.

Now, they'll say—and they have said—that "we did the best with the information we had."

No.

You.

Didn't.

And the reason I know you didn't is that, as I said before, I saw the same information and was shouting from the rooftops about what was happening, the damage we were doing. I have the receipts. I have the transcripts. And I got roundly criticized. But I was right.

Believe me, I'm not some lone genius. I didn't crack some unbreakable code. I'm not an immunologist. But I can read. And I can read people. And what I read told me that we were doing lifelong damage to our children. And, reading the people involved, I can tell you that some of them were scared of running afoul of the new consensus. Others were intoxicated by their new power: they had a new hammer and they wanted to swing it.

We saw that over and over; lots of organizations used COVID to flex their power.

I saw it personally. In Hollywood, we have union cameramen and lighting people and all sorts of other stagehands. A huge number of people depend on the film and television industries for their living— I'm talking about the people working behind the camera, not the millionaires in front of it.

So even after a vaccine was available, the unions out here wouldn't let their people come back to work without a series of COVID protocols, including a COVID compliance supervisor, which doesn't sound so unreasonable until you realize (as I have) that this person is not a medical or public health professional—the agreement that put these people in place made no mention of training or qualification.[15] They don't do the testing. They get paid thousands of dollars a week to make sure we're following the rules. So, basically a make-work job, with the job description of being a tattletale. Except in my experience, the compliance officer wasn't particularly concerned with compliance with the protocols.

And even if they had been, the protocols didn't make common sense. I appeared on a number of shows where I was required to do testing in order to feature, but the results weren't known until after the appearance. How does that protect the cast or staff at a given production? I would appear on a Monday and the results of my COVID testing would become available on Tuesday or Wednesday! The only thing those protocols allowed you to test positive for was "virtue signaling."

In the past two years, I've spent millions of dollars fulfilling these COVID protocols. We didn't need policing. Once protocols were established, everyone respected everyone else's space and compliance was uniform. It was true with my shows and every show I've visited. Because the incentive wasn't about the protocols. The real incentive was to be able to keep working, and you can't keep working if people are sick. My experience has been, if you leave things to the private sector, they will work it out. The private sector is highly incentivized to keep everyone safe and healthy so they can keep their doors open.

They don't want or need the government to come in and regulate them or shut them down.

But when people have power, it's like the old saying "You give somebody a new shovel, they're going to dig." Power is about wanting authority over people.

COVID provided an excellent opportunity for a bunch of groups to exercise their power, but that didn't mean they were exercising rational decision-making or common sense.

Because they weren't.

Prove Yourself Wrong

One final way to test rationality of thought is to prove yourself wrong.

In his famous treatise *On Liberty*, the philosopher John Stuart Mill wrote, "He who knows only his own side of the case knows little of that. His reasons may be good, and no one may have been able to refute them. But if he is equally unable to refute the reasons on the opposite side, if he does not so much as know what they are, he has no ground for preferring either opinion."

I wrote in chapter 11 that the only reason you know me is because of Oprah, and the only reason I know Oprah is because of the company I started in 1989, Courtroom Sciences Inc. (CSI).

Our company was called in to assist superlawyers Charles "Chip" Babcock and Nancy Hamilton in representing Oprah and her company Harpo Productions when she was being unjustly sued by the cattle growers up in the Texas panhandle. And the reason we were successful in defending that suit, and a whole lot of others over the years, was that we were constantly trying to *disprove ourselves*.

I like to say that nobody ever lost a case in a conference room. That's because your case sounds pretty good, your story really resonates . . . when you are the only one telling it! But, when the other side starts to pick it apart, or share *their case*, and starts filing counterclaims, it doesn't always go quite so smoothly.

So, when someone would bring us a case, the first thing we would do is argue the *other side's* position with all the vim and vigor of a mother bear protecting her cubs. We didn't even care if the opposition wasn't even in the neighborhood of logic, and in fact role-played it like our lives depended on it.

We did not tell ourselves they had a terrible case even when they did. We tried to win that position in front of a mock jury. And we usually did it way better than they ever could. In fact, sometimes we'd see the blood drain out of our clients' faces and they'd say, "I guess we need to settle this."

We'd say no, no, no, we're doing a better job on their case than they will, trust us. We just want to be ready for anything they could possibly bring. We are giving them the benefit of every doubt, assuming the judge would let in everything they wanted in, bogus or not.

We want no surprises and we want to know what we have to do to defeat the worst-case scenario. Only when we knew we could defeat the absolute best the other side could throw at us did we feel like we were ready for trial. Only then could we rationally say we had a solid and well-prepared case.

We tested our thinking.

We tested to see if what we were telling ourselves was true and believable in other people's eyes.*

There was no point in convincing *each other* that our case was factual and rational if we were the only ones who thought so.

My point is, you may have long-held beliefs that you are comfortable with and about which you have deeply entrenched feelings.

And you may be right.

---

* True and believable are key. True but not believable may give you the moral high ground, but it leaves you no better off with a jury.

You may be seeing things rationally and clearly.

What I am asking is for you to be willing to challenge *everything* in your belief system to determine if it stands up against the rationality test. If it does, then great! Hold on to that belief. But if it does not withstand challenge, don't you want to know that? If you have beliefs that are not factual, not empirically supported, wouldn't you want to know that you are embracing fictions?

If you have embraced thoughts that are not in your best interest, thoughts that are not getting you closer to what you want in your life, thoughts that do not protect and prolong your life, wouldn't you want to rid yourself of those fictions?

Irrational thoughts are self-destructive and self-defeating. They not only hold you back; they drag down the people around you. After all, the people around you are the ones who tend to like you or love you and give you the benefit of the doubt. Your irrational thinking runs the risk of leading them down a bad path.

Winners deal with the truth. Winners are very clear with themselves about the way things truly are. Instead of denying reality, they deal with reality—and they do so at the point where the outcome can still be changed.

They recognize what I'm telling you now: It doesn't matter how you feel about it, it doesn't matter how you wish it was or want it to be. Reality is what it is. Pretending it is something else because you don't like it is not rational.

Working to change it because you don't like it is something entirely different.

I'm not saying that because something is factual, or because something is empirically based, you can't find some way to change it or that you can't create a "workaround." I'm saying you can't live in a fantasy world or expect others to embrace your fiction just because you don't like the reality.

Have the courage to get real with yourself and acknowledge what is and you will have a tremendous advantage over those who con themselves and seek to con others.

If you get caught in a flood and you are the first one to acknowledge that the waters are rising, I promise you have a better chance of getting out of that situation alive than the person who pretends the waters are not rising because they wish they weren't. My dad had a philosophy that stuck with me. He said, "You better spend five percent of your time deciding whether the situation you are in is a good deal or a bad deal and ninety-five percent of your time deciding what you are going to do about it." It always made sense to me—the sooner you get to that 95 percent part, the better off you are.

Be willing to test your thinking.

Don't fall victim to confirmation bias, which distorts reality because you only see those things that confirm your belief.

You will be better for it.

Rationality is your friend.

POLL RESPONSES

How frequently do you question or measure whether your behavior patterns, projects, and pursuits in life are working or not? (This is not based on your opinion or perception, but on measurable outcomes.)

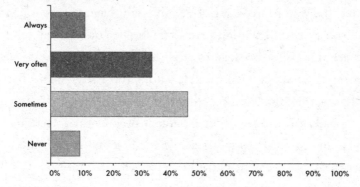

What proportion of your decisions would you say you make based on emotional reactions (versus logical or rational analysis)?

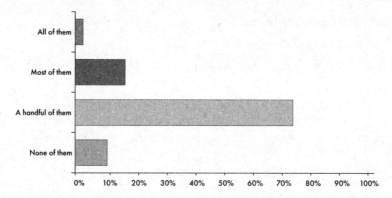

How often do you measure your outcomes based on results, and how often do you let emotions slip into your decisions? Now, we're not robots, and we don't want to be robots, but when it matters and you're dealing with things that you need to be honest with yourself about, that's when you want to deal with the truth. Denial is not your friend. You truly want to be honest with yourself.

Consciously Choose Which Voices in Your Life Deserve the Most Attention

---

POLL QUESTION

How often have you found yourself reconsidering or refusing to say what you think because you're concerned about someone else's reaction?

☐ Always

☐ Very often

☐ Sometimes

☐ Never

One of the tests I often had to administer to patients earlier in my career was the Wechsler Adult Intelligence Scale, or WAIS. The WAIS is basically an IQ test, with an emphasis on figuring out if someone can think rationally and function in society. One part of the test is verbal comprehension—do you understand what you're reading or hearing?

Part of that is exposing people to proverbs, and seeing if they understand what the lesson is. One of my favorite proverbs I've come across on the test: "Shallow brooks are noisy."

My guess is if you're reading this, you immediately understand the idea. Things that don't have depth make noise. Most people without some sort of disorder get it right away.

So, if you understand that you probably don't want to dive into a loud brook, why, in life, do we do basically the same thing? We listen to the loudest voices, without recognizing that they are often the least deserving of our attention.

And even the most credentialed people can be pretty shallow brooks sometimes.

In this world, there are an infinite number of currencies that make people light up. If you're a person of deep faith, spiritual understanding is your currency. If you're an investment banker, I'm guessing your currency is monetary currency. For drug addicts, their currency is that next hit. That's their pathway to the amygdala and that dopamine release.

> One of the key ways of understanding someone is understanding which currency is the most valuable to them. Again, I'm not talking about dollars or pesos. I'm talking about *social currency*.

One of the key ways of understanding someone is understanding which currency is the most valuable to them. Again, I'm not talking about dollars or pesos. I'm talking about *social currency*. Do they value a sense of accomplishment, and if so, how can you help them feel accomplished? And, importantly for this conversation, do they most value attention, and if so, what kind of attention?

People receive different kinds of payoffs for the things they do. If you understand what makes somebody get up in the morning and do the things they do and not do the things they don't do, then you have a really important piece of information. And let's add another key piece of information to that: for any behavior that occurs in pattern, I promise you there is a payoff.

This goes back to the famous psychologist B. F. Skinner. He

showed that our behaviors are almost entirely determined by the response we got when we demonstrated that behavior before.

So, if someone gets likes, clicks, tweets, shares, attention (positive or negative, applause or boos) for being the loudest voice, they're going to keep getting louder. All of a sudden the pursuit of attention becomes more important than thinking about what actions would actually accomplish something that would earn attention.

We know that loudmouths often compensate in volume for what they lack in wisdom. They deliver in sheer number of words what they can't accomplish with actions—as I often say, after all is said and done, usually more is said than done.

In fact, their noisiness actually gets in the way of getting things done. When you listen to the loudest voices, you're giving them the heckler's veto—the power to stop things, but not the power to accomplish things. I can give you chapter and verse on what motivates someone to be an attention-craving loudmouth blowhard. But if you're listening to them and following them without asking some key questions, then you have an issue too.

So, let's talk about why we give people and groups the attention they so desperately crave, even if they don't deserve it. And how can we stop?

Time and Attention Are Your Greatest Gifts

There's only one thing in life that you can't make more of, that you can't get back once you've given it away, and it's your time. You can make more money, but you can't make more time. Your time is your greatest gift, your most valuable offering, your nonrenewable resource.

That's why the influential pastor Rick Warren writes, "the best way to spell love is 'T-I-M-E.'"

Think about that for a bit. If time is love, how much "love" are you giving to voices or distractions that aren't worthy of it?

Because when someone or some group is asking for your attention, begging for it, screaming for it, the first question needs to be "Does this person or group deserve my time, my attention, my vote, my support?"

There are a lot of loud voices out there, and there are lots of reasons you might listen to them. Understanding those reasons is a key step in helping you live your life with intention and being who you are on purpose.

Defensive ID

Sometimes it can feel like it's not your choice to give someone your attention. One of the behaviors we see quite frequently in psychology is defensive identification. This is where someone who has been abused identifies with the person dishing out that abuse. The idea is that this is a self-protective mechanism that allows the person who is the target to avoid being targeted, avoid being cancelled, and be able to say that they belong to something.

I've seen this time and again in my work. Instead of tuning out the loud voices, we turn to them, we identify with them. We give them more of a platform.

You see it with kids who join gangs. In a lot of cases, they didn't want to be gangbangers. They saw where the strength was in their neighborhood or on their block, and so they identified with it rather than turning away or tuning out.

What If the Loudest Voice Is You?

Now I'm going to raise a sensitive subject—are you one of those voices?

For about as long as man has been able to speak, there's been assorted wisdom reminding him to occasionally shut up. In the Bible (Proverbs 17:28) we read, "Even a fool is thought wise if he keeps silent, and discerning if he holds his tongue." That's been modernized over time to various versions of "Better to keep quiet and be thought a fool than open your mouth and remove all doubt."

In fact, one of the most damning descriptions of someone I can think of is the way that Ted Sorensen, who was one of President Kennedy's closest advisors, described the CIA. "Often wrong, never in doubt."

POLL RESPONSE

How often have you found yourself reconsidering or refusing to say what you think because you're concerned about someone else's reaction?

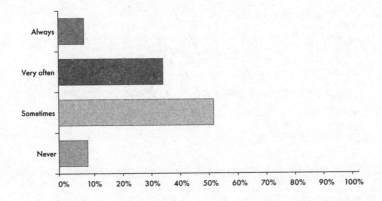

Think about that: over 90 percent of you report that you're self-censoring, and over 40 percent of you are doing it often! And as we discussed in chapter 2, not saying what you believe can actually be unhealthy for you—it causes stress and psychic pain. The reason I asked this question here is that self-censoring can be a result of fearing that you either don't want to attract the attention of the "loudest voice" or you don't have the stature or standing or authority to be heard. But guess what? You do!

Do Not Stay Silent Just So Others Can Remain Comfortable

POLL QUESTION

If someone has a negative opinion of you, how often do you let that opinion dominate your thinking or affect your life?

☐ Always

☐ Very often

☐ Sometimes

☐ Never

The First Amendment is irrelevant.

Don't get me wrong. The First Amendment may be America's greatest contribution to humanity. In less than one hundred words, it makes clear that in this country you have the freedom to say what you want, to worship how you want to worship, to gather peacefully, to ask your government to do the things that will make life better, and to have the press and the media search for the truth and hold leaders to account.

The First Amendment is what makes America America.

So why would I tell you it's irrelevant?

Because the First Amendment protects all of these rights from *government* interference.

The First Amendment offers broad protection for a large number of oral, written, and symbolic statements. (However, if you want to use your freedom of speech to defame someone, spread obscenity, commit perjury, or encourage others to commit crimes, you're out of luck.)

But the First Amendment can't protect against self-censorship, and self-censoring has become endemic. From the 1950s to today, the percentage of Americans who don't feel free to express their views has tripled. Nearly two-thirds of Americans say that today's political climate prevents them from saying things they believe because others might find them offensive.[1] More than half of college students say they feel that they can't express their opinion.[2] In fact, students are more concerned about criticism from their classmates than from their instructors.

This self-censoring doesn't only concern extreme or fringe views. Yes, conservatives are the most likely to self-censor. And yes, strong liberals are the only group where a majority feels that they can say what they believe. However, there is substantial and increasing self-censoring in every group in society.[3]

Why?

Fear.

Fear of being cancelled, boycotted, shamed, or otherwise called out for something they said in an attempt to silence them. It's become part of our culture.

There are a lot of explanations for the rise of cancel culture, but for me it comes down to two things we've discussed already in this book: belonging and power.

The number one need for people is acceptance. The number one fear is rejection. Cancellation plays to both. There's a theory called the "spiral of silence," which was coined by the political scientist Elisabeth Noelle-Neumann. The spiral-of-silence theory describes the tendency of people to muzzle themselves when they think public opinion might be against them. Going against public opinion can lead to some painful social costs and consequences. You could be criticized, scrutinized, and ostracized from your friends, family, or social groups. This leads people who judge the opinion climate to be unfavorable to their views to remain silent rather than speak out.[4]

But people cancel because they want to belong too. And what better way to belong than by gathering up a posse to go ride after the outlaw? All that's required is to identify who the outlaw is.

People constantly observe other people's behavior in order to find out which opinions and behaviors are met with approval or rejection in the public sphere. Here's where social media is like throwing gasoline on a fire, because people speak up louder and stronger when they feel public support—and I guarantee (or, actually, the algorithm guarantees) that no matter what you say, there's going to be some support coming your way. So it can escalate, fast, and to dangerous levels. One study found that when groups of people on social media believed their moral code had been violated, they felt so justified in their harassment of their targets that they refused to acknowledge it as harassment.[5]

So, who tries to cancel someone else, and why? As I said, we're all susceptible to it, because it plays into our need for belonging and our fear of rejection. But I found one study on individual motivations of people who cancel others that I think is really important to understand, because one of the motivations is *jealousy*.[6] People who become cancel targets tend to be rich, powerful, and famous. For a minute, the people attempting to bring them down can feel famous too. In that moment, the person calling for cancellation has as much power as their target. People don't feel like they have the power to change structural inequalities or deliver justice where they feel there's been an injustice done, but cancelling shows that people have an individual power to provide some sort of corrective, even if it usually ends up being a failed or misdirected one.

I have more to say about the dangers of jealousy and envy in my rule about consequential knowledge.

Cancel Culture or Consequence Culture?

I'm a big believer in consequences. I've said it time and again: you choose the behavior, you choose the consequence. You don't always have to say everything that comes to mind, and some opinions (such as racist or violent statements) should receive some backlash. Some of what we're seeing in cancel culture is that people who weren't held accountable before are being held accountable now. But when social media and public opinion are the judge, jury, and executioner, the punishment doesn't often fit the crime. What should be a discussion has instead become a tribunal.

We need a culture of public forgiveness, and maybe we have to learn to think and talk about controversial issues in a more nuanced way. We need to swap out cancel culture for a conversation culture, or a counsel culture where we can actually listen to and learn from each other. And if a person is ill-informed or misguided, someone who does have the facts, someone who does know the science can reach out to counsel the person and give them an opportunity to raise their game and develop a higher level of understanding. But if it is one-and-done, all you do is further estrange the person you cancelled. And now that person is motivated by resentment and, as we discussed in our chapter on victim culture, revenge.

> We need to swap out cancel culture for a conversation culture, or a counsel culture where we can actually listen to and learn from each other.

What a shame to create an adversary when there's a chance a different approach could have helped create a friend and supporter.

In the introduction I talked about the power of language, and how we're "catastrophizing" things that simply aren't catastrophes.

Disagreements are quickly labeled "hate speech."

We have weaponized the word *phobic*, which is what you are called when you disagree with a radical position or ask an innocent question. I can't believe I need to state something this obvious, but you are not phobic because you disagree. You are not phobic for asking a question. You may be curious. You may be doubtful. You may be lots of things, but phobic? Isn't that a huge leap that reflects "cultlike" intolerance of independent thought and a healthy, questioning attitude?

So not only are words weaponized. The *lack* of words is weaponized.

Say there's some issue out there that I really don't care all that much about. Sometimes you just don't have a dog in that race. These days that's unacceptable. You *have* to care. You *have* to speak up, because, wait for it, "silence is violence."

I am *not* a fan of this phrase. It makes no sense. Silence can indicate agreement, it can indicate disagreement, or it can indicate that I simply don't have the time for whatever you're peddling. As far as I can tell, the only thing that the phrase has going for it is that it rhymes.

Silence is not violence. Often silence is a simple statement that should be enough: I don't have anything invested here. You live your life, I'll live mine.

However, there is a set of situations in which silence is damaging—and that's when your silence is in service of a *cult of compliance*.

In 1997, Michigan State University officials received a disturbing report about Larry Nassar, who was a sports medicine physician at the school and the team doctor for USA Gymnastics. A young gymnast came forward to say that she was uncomfortable with the "intra-vaginal treatments" he was administering to her.[7] That should have been all the warning that people in positions of authority needed, because "pelvic floor physical therapy" isn't a common treatment for the type of problems that impact gymnasts. And even if it was common, it's not the doctors who usually perform the procedure—it's usually referred to a physical therapist who specializes and is certified in it, usually a woman. And whoever does the procedure, they wear gloves. Not Larry Nassar.[8]

Following that complaint, his abuse continued, and so did instances of the young women he assaulted trying to raise the alarm.

Nassar wasn't relieved of his clinical and patient duties at Michigan State for nearly two decades after that first complaint was made, and he abused hundreds of women.

Dr. James M. Heaps was another campus gynecologist and oncologist—this time at the University of California, Los Angeles. Since his arrest in 2019, hundreds of alleged victims have come forward, claiming they were sexually assaulted during one or more of their wellness examinations with Dr. Heaps. Dr. Heaps continues to maintain his innocence, and UCLA has spent about $700 million in lawsuit settlement for its role in concealing the abuse.[9] How many victims were preyed upon because others remained silent? And I'm not blaming the victims here. I'm talking about the people in power who had information from the brave patients who came forward, but who remained silent, or did their jobs slowly and grudgingly because doing their jobs would have required "speaking up." We certainly know that hundreds of additional victims came forward once the bureaucrats stepped up and did their jobs to make those who were victimized feel safe.

Not all sexual predators lurk in the shadows. Some are highly respected and trusted medical professionals working for esteemed higher institutions. They hide behind their white coats and victimize people behind the shield and shadow of their credentials and the privilege conferred by the institutions that employ them.

Now, this chapter is about the need for us to be a country where people don't stay silent in order to make other people comfortable. The people who were taken advantage of by these predators didn't stay silent. They were brave as brave can be.

We need to hold to account the corporate and institutional enablers—the administrators and bureaucrats who didn't want to rock the boat, who didn't want to risk slaughtering a cash cow.

The people who needed to speak up didn't. And that allowed a whole lot more people to get hurt.

Even after Dr. Nassar was discovered and found guilty, there were still those who wanted to add insult to injury and continue to silence the victims.

That's where Judge Rosemarie Aquilina stepped in. She allowed every woman who had been molested by Larry Nassar a chance to give a "victim impact statement" in her courtroom. A chance to look their abuser in the eye and tell him how he had hurt them. Over 150 women and girls came forward. The impact statements took days.[10]

This is what she's done in other cases as well.

She decided her courtroom was going to be a place of justice and healing. In her words, "Part of restitution means making them [victims] whole, and making them whole means that they face their devil and tell them exactly what they want so that their healing can begin."[11]

This approach wasn't without controversy. Judge Aquilina told me that she was criticized for letting her courtroom become too emotional, for letting the victim impact statements drag on for too long. Other judges felt it made them look bad, because they didn't let their courtrooms be places of emotional catharsis. But she wasn't going to remain silent for the comfort of others—not a convicted criminal and not any other judges.

The Silence of Sheepishness
(the Silence of the Lambs)

In the last chapter, about the loudest voices, I shared the old adage "Better to keep quiet and be thought a fool than open your mouth and remove all doubt." I want to recant that, in part, because you are always allowed to ask questions.

Often in life, you'll run into people who use big words or technical jargon to maintain an air of mystery, so they can assert their mastery.

How often have you had something explained to you—anything from an investment to driving directions to where in a store you can find the product you need—after which you realized, "I still have no idea what this is, or where I'm going."

(I can't tell you the number of times I've left Home Depot without what I needed because a salesperson told me where it was, I couldn't find it, and I didn't want to ask again.)

That's another definition of remaining silent so that others can be comfortable.

We're all afraid of seeming foolish or ignorant.

So, we go along even if we really don't know what we're agreeing to or where we're going.

I guarantee you, anytime you have questions, others do too.

Anything you don't understand, others don't understand.

Trying to unravel a mystery when someone else is asserting mastery can be intimidating. But your job isn't to make them comfortable. Your job is to achieve what you set out to do. And silence almost never delivers that result. Give yourself permission to go after and get the information you need to feel like you are making informed decisions. If people are threatened by your thirst for information, that's their problem. The more defensive they get, I would suggest the more they have to hide. Those who have nothing to hide, hide nothing.

And remember, peace at any price is no peace at all.

POLL RESPONSE

If someone has a negative opinion of you, how often do you let that opinion dominate your thinking or affect your life?

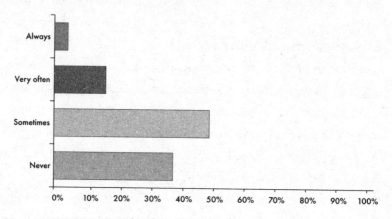

It's tough not to let someone's negative opinion of you intrude into your thinking. And so we often don't want to "tempt negativity" by speaking up. But you'd be surprised how often your willingness to speak up will create a positive response among others who have felt similarly silenced.

Now I don't want to mislead you here. I'm not saying that speaking up may not come at a price, because those who want you to stop talking, to stop asking questions, may try to punish you in order to silence you. But you've got to decide whether you're going to be who you are on purpose, or if you're going to let someone else paddle your boat. I think the positives to speaking up definitely outweigh the negatives.

Actively Live and Support a Meritocracy

POLL QUESTIONS

How often do you encounter someone who you believe got their job because of some unfair advantage?

- ☐ Always
- ☐ Very often
- ☐ Sometimes
- ☐ Never

How often do you interact with someone who you know got their job for a reason other than their skill or knowledge?

- ☐ Always
- ☐ Very often
- ☐ Sometimes
- ☐ Never

I'm sure you've heard a million times that one of America's big problems is income inequality—that the gap between rich and poor is growing too large, and that capitalism just isn't working.[1]

But what if I told you that one of the biggest problems in our country isn't income inequality, it's *income equality*—that we've set up a system where people who are working hard to get by barely make more money than people who aren't working at all. Well, that's exactly what's happening.

Let me explain. John Early, who helped run the Bureau of Labor Statistics, and Phil Gramm, who used to lead the US Senate Banking Committee, took a look at the numbers and found that if you take all of the incomes in America and divide them into five groups, the bottom group earned just under $7,000 a year on average. And only a little more than a third of them were employed.

The second group, one step up, earned $31,800 on average, and 85 percent of them were employed. That's America: work harder, earn more, climb your way up. But I think if we're being honest, it's barely possible to support yourself on $7,000 a year and damn near impossible to raise a family on $31,000.

So, your government makes what are called "transfer payments" to people in this country who don't earn much income. Those payments take a lot of forms. Tax credits. Welfare. Medicaid. And nearly one hundred other government programs.[2] These payments to that second group, which earns $31,000 on average, has the effect of bumping up their income to just over $50,000. That's a hand up. You're working, but you're not making enough to get by, and we help you out.

But what about the folks at the bottom who mostly aren't working and are earning $7,000 on average? Well, they also get transfer payments and tax breaks. And you know that those add up to? Nearly $49,000 a year, almost exactly the same as the person who is working and making $31,000 a year.

You're probably saying, that doesn't sound right. If I can make as much money by not working as I can by working, not working sounds like a pretty good deal. And that's exactly what has happened—a lot of folks checked out of the labor force.

And it's not just the bottom two groups. Let's look at the middle group of earners—these are folks making about $66,000 a year. More than 90 percent of them work, and because they pay taxes and don't get many "transfers," they keep, on average, just over $61,000. That's just 26 percent more than the bottom quintile. So about 60 percent of

Americans are all taking home basically the same amount of money, even though there are massive variations in how much and how hard they work.

That's not too much wealth inequality. That's too much *equality*. That's government not only taking away the will to work. That's government taking away self-determination. That's government saying that we're going to have equality of outcomes, even if there's no quality of inputs. And that's a problem. Knowledge should differentiate you. Hard work should differentiate you. Skill should differentiate you. That's economy-wide. But it's happening in every part of our lives too—with disastrous consequences.

We're Seeing It Everywhere

One of the biggest scandals in our country today is how organizations across the board are dropping standards to match the proficiency levels of the people they have. I'm talking about colleges, police departments, even pools are dropping the qualification for lifeguards!

In chapter 2, I mentioned that when Michael Eisner, who was CEO of Disney at the time, was being wheeled in for emergency heart surgery, he called his wife over to ask about the doctor who was scheduled to do his surgery. "Where was this guy trained?" he asked. In his book he wrote, "She knew I was hoping to hear Harvard or Yale. 'Tijuana,' she replied, with a straight face."[3]

Why is this story funny? Because this big-shot CEO wanted to know that he was under the care of the best. When you go into a doctor's office, there are all sorts of diplomas and certifications on the wall. They tell you: this person is qualified.

But they only tell you that if they *mean something*. If they mean that you passed the most rigorous training, did the hardest work, out-worked, out-thought, out-studied everyone else. What you don't want those diplomas and certificates to mean is: We gave this person this certification because they were oppressed. Or we had a quota to fill. Or we felt bad for them because they were having a hard time that semester.

One of my friends quotes some wisdom he received from a track coach: "Nobody cares less about your ego than a stopwatch." Results matter.

Now, I'm not one who believes that fancy-pants schools produce the best people. My journey took me through the University of Tulsa, Texas Tech University, Midwestern State University, North Texas State—and I am proud of the teaching and training I received at each of those places.

I met some of the smartest people I'll ever have the honor of knowing at those places. A lot of them were first in their families to go to college. So, I don't need to see a Harvard or a Yale on your diploma—heck, I don't really need to see any diploma at all, so long as I know you did the work and got to where you are by the sweat of your brow and the brain that's behind it.

In fact, I've had a lot of Harvard lawyers working for me over the years, and a lot of them were really book smart but didn't have the common sense or life experience to order lunch. You could put them in the back office with a stack of law books and they could brief the heck out of something, but they couldn't try a case if you held a gun on them.

These days we're sacrificing skill and talent on the altar of feelings and quotas. And I'm telling you, that's going to bite everyone in the butt. In some places, it already has.

So, when Michael Eisner wanted to make sure he was getting the best, I realize you don't need to be a big-time CEO to feel that way. It doesn't need to be heart surgery. I don't want to get on a plane where the pilot isn't the best trained. I don't want to be represented by a lawyer who doesn't know their stuff. You don't want a tire changed on the car you'll be using to drive yourself or your children by someone not competent to have put the tire and wheel safely back on your car.

These days we're sacrificing skill and

talent on the altar of feelings and quotas. And I'm telling you, that's going to bite everyone in the butt. In some places, it already has.

Let me give you a few examples.

Lowering Standards in the Classroom[4]

Meet Maitland Jones Jr. He's an experimental chemist and a professor. He teaches, or, rather, he taught, a course on organic chemistry, first for many years at Princeton University, and then, after retiring from there, at New York University. You'd be hard-pressed to find someone more qualified to do the job. He literally wrote the book—the textbook, that is—on organic chemistry, 1,300 pages and now in its fifth edition. He received awards for his teaching and was recognized as one of NYU's coolest professors by OneClass, a place where students can share class notes and study guides.[5]

Now, if you have any scientists or doctors in your family, they'll be the first to tell you that organic chemistry is a nightmare, a really hard course. And it's supposed to be. For decades it has served as a "weed out" class, meaning that it is intended to be difficult by design, a hurdle that only the most serious students can clear.

That's the whole point of it.

As the students at OneClass noted, "Orgo is a nightmare, and Maitland, who wrote the Orgo textbook, an internationally renowned experimental chemist and avid jazz lover, can actually make it a nightmare as well. But it's really just tough love: Maitland will push you to understand Organic chemistry radically and you will come out of his course having the best tools to use to become a chemist."

But Dr. Jones started to notice something a while ago. In an interview with the *New York Times*, he said that "he noticed a loss of focus among the students, even as more of them enrolled in his class, hoping to pursue medical careers."[6]

He said that "students were misreading exam questions at an astonishing rate." Even though he made exams less difficult, student grades continued to fall. Dr. Jones attributed some of this to the COVID pandemic and the learning loss associated with it. So, paying his own money, and with a couple of other professors, he videotaped fifty-two of his chemistry lectures—so that students could access them at any time.

But student performance still went down. As Dr. Jones said, "They weren't coming to class, that's for sure, because I can count the house. They weren't watching the videos, and they weren't able to answer the questions."

What the students were doing, however, was complaining.

They complained that the professor's tone was "condescending and demanding."

They argued that a class with so many low grades doesn't make the students look bad: it makes the chemistry department and NYU look bad.

NYU tried to calm the students down by offering them the chance to withdraw from the class after the fact, so a bad or failing grade wouldn't show up on their record.

The head of the chemistry department called this a "gentle but firm hand to the students and those who pay the tuition bills." I would call it something else—coddling.

But even that wasn't enough. In 2020, 82 of the 350 students in the class signed a petition saying, "We are very concerned about our scores, and find that they are not an accurate reflection of the time and effort put into this class."

And what did NYU do? They terminated Dr. Jones's contract. One of the most distinguished professors in his field, a man whom the majority of the students in his class defended and admired, was fired.

A former chairman of the department summed it up this way: "He hasn't changed his style or methods in a good many years. The students have changed, though, and they were asking for and expecting more support from the faculty when they're struggling."[7]

After all this, several students told the *Washington Post* that they never intended to get Jones fired; they just wanted better grades.[8] Last I checked, the way to get better grades is to do the work. Attend the lectures. Get extra help if you need it. And if you still can't get the material, maybe you need to find a different path. There's no shame in that; it's part of the journey toward finding your consequential knowledge, as I discuss in the next chapter.

Look, I love the wonderful surprises like when my friend Oprah gets to tell everyone in her audience, "You get a car, and you get a car." But what if she had said, "You get to be a doctor! And you get to be a doctor!" We would be saying, "Hold on a second, I'm not sure I want you to be *my* doctor." There would be less cheering in that studio audience.

By the way, I invited Dr. Jones to come on my show, and he respectfully declined. He just didn't want to talk about it anymore, and I get it. This guy has been beaten up, maligned, and made an example of, all because he did one of the most noble things in the world—he chose to teach the next generation, he had the gall to push them to be better and made the career-ending mistake of telling them when they were falling short and had to do better.

When that becomes a firing offense, you can see why I fear for our country and our future.

Now, some look at this story and say there's no reason for "weed out" culture—that passing a tough organic chemistry course doesn't have much to do with whether you can be a good doctor. Fine. I'm happy to have that conversation. Until then, don't lower the bar on what has been a key part of the training of every doctor in this country and helped us develop the most advanced biomedical industry in the world.

How did the most foundational, American belief somehow become the most controversial? Maybe because we think merit is not assessed fairly.

We expect people to win the race, but they have to have a track to run on. And some people never got on the track. No matter how hard they might be willing to work, they don't get a fair shot. That may be true, and that needs to go high on the to-do list. However, that doesn't mean that I want to go into open-heart surgery and have less than the best working on me. If there's a brilliant heart surgeon to be, figure out a way to get them on the track. Until then, I don't want someone operating on me who couldn't pass organic chemistry. You're not going to solve any problems by taking someone who is not qualified and giving them the job. You're not going to solve the problem of diversity among our nation's pilots by lowering admissions or grading standards at the airline pilots' academy. That's not fair to anybody, because you're setting people up to fail.

You have to fix unfairness earlier on in the process. And until we do, I'm going to continue to strongly advocate for a 100 percent meritocracy and indict the woke mentality that we should lower the bar so that more people can clear it, or because we're responding to some sort of social agenda, guilt, or any agenda other than skill, performance, and ability.

Consider the college admissions process. You can't fix inequality at the college admissions level if you don't fix it at the elementary school level. It's like the surgery I recently had on my knee. I needed a full replacement because you can't fix the top without also fixing the bottom—otherwise you've just moved the pain to a different location. And when I did a full fix, I wanted the best of the best, not someone given the job so the hospital could "virtue signal" its commitment to diversity.

As I was working on this book, the United States Supreme Court agreed—outlawing affirmative action based on race in college admissions. The court said that applicants should be judged on their merits as individuals, not as members of the racial group they belong to.

Part of the problem with giving advantages to "groups" is that not every individual reflects the characteristics of the group. There are plenty of rich Black and Hispanic families in this country who send their children to elite schools and have as many advantages and as much privilege as any rich white person. Should they get additional advantages? And there are a lot of poor white kids who are struggling to lift themselves up through education. Should they be further disadvantaged?

This focus on "group" over "individual" has also infected the corporate world through a philosophy known as DEI—diversity, equity, and inclusion. Companies institute these programs to hire employees from underrepresented racial groups.[9] But there's that word again—*groups*. We all bring different individual experiences and perspectives to our jobs. We want diverse perspectives—that's a good thing, it helps teams better understand challenges, solve problems, and connect with customers. But that comes from diverse individuals, not group quotas.

In case you think the result of these court decisions or the backlash against DEI is fewer opportunities for certain minorities, I want to be totally clear on this point. Meritocracy means meritocracy, and another group that is really going to feel disadvantaged by a meritocracy—and will be—is the unqualified kid who gets into a fancy college because their parents went there, or their grandparent's family name is on the library. I don't want a legacy pilot or a legacy surgeon, either. If they are fully qualified, fine. They shouldn't be excluded because of a legacy, but they should have to meet the standard just like everyone else.

I don't want Hunter Biden or Donald Trump Jr. doing squat for me if they didn't earn the right by demonstrating competencies. Heck, if someone has a roman numeral after their name, color me suspicious.

Our refusal to accept the core American tenet of meritocracy shows up both in places that are silly and those that are deadly serious.

Lowering Standards Is a Life-or-Death Issue

Here's one example: to be a lifeguard at a New York City pool or beach, you're supposed to be able to swim four hundred yards in just under seven minutes for the beach, and just under eight minutes for a pool. Those are high standards. They're not easy to meet. And that's okay, because these people are *lifeguards*.

In 2022, New York City faced a lifeguard shortage, so they changed the rules for lifeguards in the smallest pools. Now they only need to be able to swim three hundred yards, with no time restriction.[10] Big difference.

Now, these people are only allowed to guard pools that are three feet deep, so they'll never really need to swim at all, so this probably won't make much of a difference. But someone designed those initial standards *for a reason*. And if we're going to lower those standards, it should be for a reason too. A reason other than "not enough people could meet the initial standard."

As I'm writing this, our country has just watched the video of the brutal police beating and, I think it's safe to call it, murder of Tyre Nichols in Memphis, Tennessee. I'm not going to go into the specifics of that case or the officers involved. But I will say this: something like this was bound to happen sooner or later, because Memphis lowered their standards for what it takes to be a police officer.

Alvin Davis was a lieutenant in charge of recruiting for the Memphis Police Department. He retired in 2022 out of frustration, and here's what he said: "They would allow just pretty much anybody to be a police officer because they just want these numbers."

And the facts support his claim. The department got rid of the requirements that were previously needed to become a police officer—college credits, military service, or previous police work. The department petitioned the state to give them the freedom to hire applicants with criminal records. (In fact, one of the officers who killed Tyre Nichols had an arrest record himself. Another had a history of violence that probably would have gotten his application denied if there were more qualified applicants to be had.)

The academy got rid of timing requirements on physical fitness drills. They removed running entirely, because too many people were failing. Do you know what's required to be a Memphis police officer right now? Two years of work experience. Any work experience.

According to the Associated Press, one former patrol officer who became a recruiter said, "In addition to drawing from other law enforcement agencies and college campuses, recruits were increasingly coming from jobs at the McDonald's and Dunkin' drive-thrus."[11]

In one case, a stripper with an arrest record applied to be a police officer. She didn't get the job, and that's probably a good thing—because you don't want to be blurring the line between "stripper dressed as a police officer" and "stripper who is also a police officer."

I said this was about two issues. One is lowering standards. The other is installing quotas. Both are wrong.

I spend a lot of time in Hollywood and I see it happening in entertainment. Ask anyone in Hollywood—anyone—and they'll tell you privately (but they won't say publicly) that unless their project meets certain quotas—people of color, gay people, transgender people—in front of and behind the camera, it's not getting made.

Casting is under pressure not to choose the best actors for the role, or actors who can help make the project a financial success, but to make sure that "representation" comes first and foremost.

Actors are getting condemned for playing roles outside their background, upbringing, or ethnicity—getting accused of appropriating from others. Directors are getting cancelled for it.

The singer Sia was excited to direct her first movie, called *Music*, about an autistic teenager named, appropriately, Music. To play the lead character, Sia cast an actor named Maddie Ziegler, who is not autistic. In today's wordsmith terminology, Maddie Ziegler is "neurotypical."

Cancel culture went crazy, with one Twitter user expressing a view that the internet came to embrace: "It's a mighty shame that someone with such a colossal platform is using it to exclude disabled and neuro diverse actors from their own narratives."[12]

Sia responded by pointing out that she actually had cast the film in a very diverse way. "I cast thirteen neurotypical people, three trans folk, and not as f——-ing prostitutes or drug addicts but as doctors, nurses and singers."

In fact, Sia had tried to cast an autistic actor in the lead role, but the actor found it unpleasant and stressful. In other words, in this case, the autistic actor couldn't do that job. Sia felt that it was more compassionate—and would help others feel more compassion— to cast the actor she ultimately did cast, fourteen-year-old Maddie Ziegler.

The controversy got so heated that Ziegler was reduced to tears, worried that people would say her performance was insensitive.

Which brings up another point. This whole controversy erupted before anyone had actually seen the movie. Choose sides! Tear Sia down! Cancel! I can tell you that nobody reached their own conclusion because nobody could have reached their own conclusion—they hadn't seen the movie.

If they had, they would have seen a performance that Steven Spielberg said was fantastic. They would have seen a movie that the Child Mind Institute had fully approved as being sensitive to the autism community.

Amid the controversy, Sia pointed out something else.

"There is no way I could have used someone of [Music's] level of functioning to play her. . . . I also needed a dancer, for [the character's] imaginary life. It's not a documentary. Kate [Hudson, who play's Music's half sister] isn't a drug dealer and Leslie Odom Jr. [who plays Ebo] isn't from Ghana."[13]

She said it better than I could. Acting is ACTING!! You PLAY someone else. That's what acting is! You aren't appropriating. Tom Hanks said he wouldn't do the movie *Philadelphia* if it were today because he isn't gay! In his words, "We are beyond that now." But what if a gay man doesn't want to come out yet? What if there is not an equal talent available among gay actors?

Helen Mirren took a lot of heat for playing the late Israeli prime minister Golda Meir, even though she's not Jewish. Mirren asked the right question there too, saying, "If someone who's not Jewish can't play Jewish, does someone who's Jewish play someone who's not Jewish?"[14]

Ana de Armas took heat for being a Cuban woman playing Marilyn Monroe. Come on! She won the role.

Are transgender actors only going to play transgender roles? If they play straight roles are they appropriating? This has gone nuts.

Diversity and inclusion are now defined as staying in one's own lane?

One of the things my son Jay has done very effectively is help inform younger people about their health. As Jay writes in his book *The Ultimate Weight Solution for Teens*, "Weight is not about the size of your Levis or a number on the scale. It's about whether you use food to take care of your body or to abuse it."

As part of his research process, Jay went out in the world wearing a "fat suit" to gain insight into how overweight people are discriminated against. It was an eye-opening experience for him and for all of us. He was basically dismissed from a job interview when he was in the suit, and straight-up offered the job when he wasn't. I suspect today an investigation like that would be criticized by the "everybody is a victim culture," without any thought given to the fact that it was powerfully effective at exposing the unfairness overweight people endure. But, when the only tool you have is a hammer, everything looks like a nail. (I'm sure that somehow offends hammers.)

POLL RESPONSES

How often do you encounter someone who you believe got their job because of some unfair advantage?

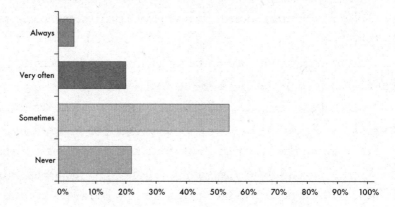

How often do you interact with someone who you know got their job for a reason other than their skill or knowledge?

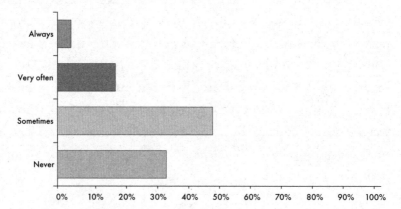

At first glance, these two questions may seem to be the same, but they're not. First of all, you can't always know why someone else got a job, or a role, or a position. Remember, we live our lives reacting not to what happened, but to the stories we *tell ourselves* about what happened. So the difference between "believe" (in the first question) and "know" (in the second question) is a big one.

Similarly, there's a distinction between an "unfair advantage" and " a reason other than skill or knowledge." The difference in the questions led to slightly more "doubt" in your responses to the second one. In both cases, however, the result may be unfair to you. But remember, it's also unfair to the person who got the job. Either they've been set up to fail, or they have to labor under your suspicion (and everyone else's) that they're there for the wrong reason.

Identify and Build Your Consequential Knowledge

POLL QUESTION

Are you comfortable that you have identified, developed, and continue to develop that skill or talent that puts you in the best position in a competitive marketplace?

☐ Totally comfortable

☐ Very comfortable

☐ Somewhat comfortable

☐ Not comfortable

Back in early 2000s, there was a popular TV show called *The Wire*, which followed various aspect of life in the city of Baltimore—the police, the schools, and, in the second season, the ports.

There's murder and crime and bribes, of course. But, to me, the most powerful scene is when one of the stevedores—the guys who load and unload the ships—sees a video of a fully automated port in Europe. He calls it a "horror movie . . . robots, piers full of robots. My kid will be lucky if he's even punching numbers [moving shipping containers] five years from now."

I would put that character's fear in slightly different terms. He was afraid that he and his son did not have—or at least in the future would not continue to have—what I call *consequential knowledge*.

What is consequential knowledge?

Consequential knowledge is something that you are mastering or have mastered that the rest of the world perceives to constitute added value to the world, at least to their world. As a result, it is something they are willing to pay you for. And I don't necessarily mean pay you in dollars and cents. I mean pay you in whatever form of currency you value, as I discuss under Rule #5, about the loudest voices.

Consequential knowledge is something you have to offer that the world wants and is willing to reward you for. But that's not the only set of rewards consequential knowledge provides.

When *you* observe *you* doing whatever embodies your consequential knowledge and when you experience the world rewarding you for it, that helps you feel good about yourself as a contributing member of society. It's that set of transactions that can cause you to attribute to yourself "mastery" over that domain. You might say things to yourself like "These people, this company, this community need me. Without me, without what I bring to the group, something would be missing, I would be missed. *I matter*." In this way, consequential knowledge contributes to building rock-solid self-esteem and self-worth.

And more likely than not, consequential knowledge also results in monetary worth.

That character in that show I just mentioned may have been right. For a lot of jobs, robots really are the horror movie.

Right now, in the United States, there are about 3.3 million truck drivers. It's not easy work, but truckers can earn good money. Having a specialized license is a skill. In fact, truckers are in demand. But it's now estimated that self-driving trucks could replace about 500,000 long-haul trucking jobs in the US.[1] And think about the trickle-down effects. Robots won't stop at truck stops to eat or sleep. So those jobs go away too. They won't wear boots or hats or gloves or pants or shirts. Lots of support jobs will be lost, and those folks will need to retrain and find new consequential knowledge. (By the way, it's not a total horror movie yet. The new technologies will take a while to work beyond the open road. Driving in busier, more populated settings is still a specialized skill. As are all the other jobs truckers do, like loading and unloading, customer service, actually responding to warning lights like low tire pressure or an unbalanced load. And then in the future, one of the job areas expected to grow are the people who program and repair the technologies that will be doing the driving, but you get my point.)[2]

Or look at call centers—in the industry, they're called "contact centers." Roughly 3 million Americans work in contact centers.[3] But the industry believes that they can save $80 billion by having more of the job done by artificial intelligence (AI).

Now, if you've had any interaction on the phone with an automated response robot, you know the technology isn't there yet—not even close. I can't tell you the number of times Robin has heard me shouting, "Agent, please, agent!" into the phone. But with that much savings on the line, AI is going to get there.

In fact, it's estimated that automation could eliminate 73 million jobs by 2030—whether those jobs are driving cars or flipping burgers or even writing software code.[4] Machines and technology have made farming so efficient that it requires many fewer people to grow and harvest the food we depend on. In 1900, roughly 40 percent of the total US population lived on farms. Today it's 1 percent.[5]

It's terrifying. It's demoralizing. By some estimates, nearly 40 percent of all Americans live in fear of automation coming for their jobs.

Consequential knowledge is the antidote to this fear. It's a necessary characteristic of what defines you that will allow you to take ownership of your life and future.

This isn't about having to become a software expert or a brain surgeon (robots are coming for both of those jobs too). This isn't about getting a fancy degree and going from blue collar to white collar.

It's about knowing exactly what you can offer this world.

It doesn't need to be some rare or unique skill.

It just needs to be something where you can't be replaced in two hours.

If you are a copier repairman or can fix an HVAC system—that's consequential knowledge.

They can't replace you by noon.

If you want to get ahead in this world, you need to identify what your aptitudes are and you need to develop *your* consequential knowledge. If you don't, you're a face in the crowd. You are a bit player, and you're not going to star in your own life.

If you want to star in your own life, then be a star: find out what you're good at, develop that vertically, and take pride in that consequential knowledge. What do I mean by "develop that vertically"? On a scale of zero to 100, instead of developing a skill level of 10 or 15 in seven or eight areas, I'm saying you should pick one area, one skill set, one talent and develop *vertically* in that specific area. Work your way up that scale toward 100 in proficiency; get *really good* at least at one skill or talent the world sees as added value. Choose wisely. I would not want to be the repairman for the folding door on phone booths! When was the last time you even saw a pay phone?

Understand I'm not saying you shouldn't learn as much as you can about as many things as possible. Of course you should. But you don't

> **If you want to get ahead in this world, you need to identify what your aptitudes are and you need to develop *your* consequential knowledge. If you don't, you're a face in the crowd. You are a bit player, and you're not going to star in your own life.**

want to be just a "jack of all trades, master of none," you want multiple areas of competency, but it's important to be *really* exceptional at one thing. So good, so essential at that one thing you will be missed if you're not there. You need people to need what you have to offer for things to go well.

For years, Robin and I have had a friend who is a carpenter named Marvin. He came to this country from Guatemala, and initially he took jobs here and there, doing different things.

But he realized that he loved working with wood. He loved the smell of sawdust. He loved the pride he felt with everything he created—and he took pictures of every project he completed. And then, when he started to get hired for his work, he developed himself vertically. He didn't say, "Sure, I can do plumbing or electrical too." That would have been horizontal development. Horizontal development is like when you go to a diner, and the menu is thirty-eight pages long and you think, "If they've got spaghetti and meatballs, and tacos and seafood, they might be able to do everything, but they probably aren't the best at anything. They've gone too horizontal." That's why, when you want pasta, you go to an Italian place, and when you want tacos you go to a Mexican place, and when you want fish you go to a seafood place. That's the power of vertical knowledge.

So Marvin could have been a handyman and done a little bit of everything.

But he decided to be an artisan, and carpentry was his consequential knowledge—that was the horse he was going to ride. So he continued to do more and more sophisticated woodworking. Robin showed him a drawing of a dining room table she envisioned. To say it was elaborate and intricate would be a huge understatement. I couldn't have figured out where to even try to buy this thing, never mind build it. But Marvin took one look and his mind started working. He and Robin were sketching and designing, and he was bringing in samples of wood and wood patterns, and experimenting with different finishes. Before long, he built something that incorporated all of her ideas, but ended up even more beautiful than even she had imagined. He is narrowly, vertically developed as a cabinet and finish carpenter and because of that, he can't be replaced. Better yet (for him, and sometimes—ouch—for me) he can charge a premium.

Interestingly, his brother has followed the same example, and does the painting and finishes. He can paint Sheetrock so beautifully you'll think you're walking down a hallway made of marble. He is just as amazing at what he does. Fueled by pride and passion and hard work, they both went all in. Individually and together, they are consequential to dozens and dozens of decorating and painting projects, small to massive. Always busy, always happy.

These are guys who grew up living on dirt floors in Guatemala. I asked them what they did when it rained. Their answer was, "We found pavement." They could have seen themselves as victims. Instead they've developed their consequential knowledge and made good livings and built good lives.

How many people out there have great talent and great skill that they never discover or tap into because they don't follow through? They're sitting there, whining that they're a victim, instead of exploring the depth of their talent, skill, and ability. Do you know anyone who fits that description? I'm betting you do.

Alfred E. Kahn, who is known for deregulating America's airlines, began his career as an economist. He often told the story of his time as dean at Cornell University. At one point, a bunch of English professors came to him and said, "Why are the economics professors getting paid more?" And he said, "When you can set up a profitable 'English consulting firm,' come talk to me."

His point was that the economics professors had consequential knowledge that was valuable to the school *and* on the open market.

Now, I want to be clear: I'm in a profession where my consequential knowledge is analysis and communication. Like a carpenter, people in my profession have tools we use. Our tools go by names like standardized psychometrics, if you are a diagnostician. Those tools can be put to use in lots of ways, in areas as diverse as deception detection, reading body language, learning how to help individuals and groups overcome self-destructive tendencies, and how to defuse a potentially violent or suicidal situation, to name a few.

There is a science to human behavior, no doubt. But when we are done with our work for the day there is no bridge to marvel at, no car to drive, no house to move into. I don't make or build anything. I like to think I help heal psyches, marriages, and sometimes communities and businesses. But nothing I do is broken on an x-ray when I start or healed on the x-ray when I finish.

People pay me to think and talk. When you think about it, that can be kind of a scary way to go through life, really. Robin has always joked and said, "Maybe you should wear a helmet." It was funny until I fell down a spiral staircase last summer and almost broke my neck and split my head open like a melon!

Robin, ever the source of kindness and compassion, reminded me that if I damage my brain, we're screwed. We may be screwed anyway, because I don't think she has really weighed what the impact of artificial intelligence (AI) will be as it pertains to me.

I'm not even joking. AI programs learn from the input they are "fed." The more information an AI platform can access, the more efficient it is at a task relevant to the input. Well, I've inadvertently "fed" these platforms quite a lot. I have about four thousand hours of television doing what I do. I have nine books (plus workbooks) talking about what I talk about. That's thousands of pages. When all of that focused input gets put into an AI platform that can process faster and has better recall than any human ever could . . . well, let's just say, I'd *better* keep reinventing myself, or wearing a helmet won't help!

So, for our own fulfillment and our own survival, we need to keep discovering, developing, rediscovering, and then redeveloping our consequential knowledge. That's the only way to achieve the outcome we want.

So, when people say they want an equal outcome in life, I don't even know how to interpret that. What, I ask myself, do they really want? If everyone is starving and hopeless, does being equally hungry and lost constitute an equal outcome? If everybody meets the "3 H's"—Hungry, Hopeless, Homeless—have we achieved equality? Everybody happy now?

Or are they *really* looking for something different? As in a redistribution of wealth? I find that the people who trumpet equality the loudest are looking to have their circumstances improved in a way that isn't proportionate to their contributions.

They're looking at a life they don't have and saying, "That's what I want to be equal to! I may not need the mansion. I'm not saying I wouldn't take it, but I just want you to sell it and give me the difference between what I have and what I wish I had."*

My response is a list of questions:

What is your consequential knowledge?

What are you doing to identify and then develop consequential knowledge?

What are you willing to do to create and pursue a path to consequential knowledge?

I believe in helping those who help themselves. That is not just a cliché. As I said earlier, I believe there is a huge difference between a "hand up" and a "handout." That's not just a cliché either.

Not everyone has an equal opportunity, and we all need to work to level the playing field *not* by lowering standards but by increasing

---

* Look, I believe that anyone who works hard and plays by the rules should always have what they need. I'm not talking about needs here; I'm talking about wishes.

opportunities to get those who are not prepared for the next level to get prepared for that next level.

I hear people say, "Tax the rich!" I even saw a liberal member of Congress wear a designer dress with those words printed on it (ironically, she was wearing it to one of the most lavish New York social events of the year) and I thought, "You have got to be kidding me. Especially when you look at their definition of *who* is rich!" I realize that I am not objective here. By any definition they use, I would be considered *rich*. How did I get that way? Well, I did not inherit anything from my father but a stack of bills and a mother to care for (which I was beyond happy to do!).

I worked hard and paid my way to a good education. And kept working hard and have employed hundreds and hundreds of equally hardworking people, many of them with families, generating billions of dollars of economic impact in my communities.

I have paid my taxes and supported charities.

And they want to target me and a lot of entrepreneurial folks just like me?

Now, as I'm writing this book, I am reading about a proposal that probably also targets you. Under this plan, borrowers looking to buy a home would pay higher fees for having a higher credit score. Usually having a higher credit score means it's less risky to lend money to you, so why would someone propose that those borrowers should have higher fees? Because that money would then go to subsidize borrowers who have lower credit scores.[6] What an absolute slap in the face to those home loan applicants who lived within their means to establish a good credit rating and one day benefit from a lower rate and lower mortgage fees. How insane is this, that the person who has a solid application gets less favorable terms than the person standing next to you who files a weaker application?

Equal outcomes don't make sense in a world of unequal inputs.

You Are the CEO of You

In the early 1960s, a vice president of the Frito Company (which later became Frito-Lay) named Arch West was vacationing with his family in Southern California. They decided to grab a bite to eat at a roadside shack, where Arch and his family were served a fried corn chip that had a tangy seasoning on it.[7]

Arch thought that this could be a whole new product, at a time when Americans were starting to sample new flavors. His bosses weren't enthusiastic. So he secretly funneled some budget money from other departments to do a little research and development on his snack idea. After testing the new product in California and getting a good response, the product went national. Its name? Doritos. Doritos became Frito's second-bestselling brand (behind potato chips), and the world buys billions of dollars of them a year.

Taking a risk, inventing a new product—none of these were in Arch's job description. But he had consequential knowledge, he knew about people's changing tastes. He knew what they liked to eat (he had previously worked doing marketing for Jell-O).[8]

When Arch died in 2011, his family tossed some Doritos into the grave as tribute. As his daughter said, "He would think it is hilarious."[9] I think it's a perfect tribute to a guy who recognized that he might have been the vice president of a big company, but he was the CEO of himself.

I tell you that, to tell you this: I don't care where you work or what you do, at some level you are in business for yourself. You are a company of one. You are the CEO of "YOU, Inc."

So, I want you to pitch me on YOU, Inc.!

Tell me, do you *believe* in YOU, Inc.?

Are you passionate about YOU?

Do you have an annual plan for your company?

Are you setting goals?

Are you positioning your company to achieve what you want to come to pass?

I recognize that you are not technically a small business, but it's worth noting that about 50 percent of small businesses fail in the first five years. The reasons vary, but lack of preparation and refusing to deviate from a failed business model certainly make the list.

So, if you're a small business, the statistics tell you that survival requires being better than the bottom half. And as you're surviving, you'd better be learning.

The same is true for YOU, Inc. Don't be stubborn: adapt. Especially if your business model isn't working. You can't fire you! So you need to get along with you and make things work. Despite what some people, often *loud* people, might tell you, this country *is* a meritocracy.

It rewards hard work and persistence. And it is a meritocracy that is also a *capitalist* society, which means that hard work and persistence can yield real gains. Now, we can debate whether that is a good thing or a bad thing (although, to my mind, there's no debate at all; history proves that socialism does not work), but you can argue about different economic systems until you are blue in the face, and when you are done with the debate, America will still be a merit-based system that rewards hard work, creativity, and results.

So, my advice is this: work hard, stay after your goals. Misery and complaint are not a strategy.

Your Consequential Knowledge Is a Shield

When I was doing my training in psychology, I had a few professors who just did not like me, hard as that may be to believe! One woman in particular, who was in a position of power, just seemed to have it out for me. I was already published, which I think she resented. I drove a nice car and already had business interests. I just don't think I fit her expectation of "grad student," which in her mind meant "subservient."

She probably would have busted me out of the program if she could. But she couldn't afford to get rid of me because I was a top student with top scores and I had the support of the entire rest of the faculty. I was a teaching assistant, helped represent the program to the certification committees that made visits to evaluate our program, and got a first-call internship placement. She didn't like me, but it didn't matter. I protected myself by being the type of student—and the type of academic story—that they needed. Having consequential knowledge fortifies you. It inoculates you from arbitrary victimization. Make yourself as indispensable as you can.

Success Leaves Clues

I've studied success for a long, long time, and it leaves clues. It's not an accident. People don't succeed by accident. In fact, when people *do* succeed by accident—like by winning the lottery, or lucking into a promotion they didn't deserve—they usually unsucceed pretty quickly, either by going bankrupt or failing at their job. Meanwhile, if you study some people who are successful, whether it's in athletics, or teaching, or business, or medicine, you will find there is a pattern.

First, successful people know what they want. They know what success is. They know what it will look like when they achieve it.

They may be falsely modest. They may say, "Oh, I don't want to talk about my success and jinx myself." But privately and often publicly, the true champions will say, "I know exactly what success looks like. I know how it's going to feel, how it's going to look, how it's going to smell, who's going to be there, what I'm going to be wearing."

If you ask a football player what it's going to be like if they win the Super Bowl, they can tell you exactly how it's going to feel when those final seconds tick off the clock. It's like they have developed muscle memory for something that hasn't happened yet. They know it. They can sense it. They can feel it. Their personal truth tells them they deserve it.

And that's important because, second, they take action toward a known outcome. I'll say it again: successful people take action toward a known outcome. It's like the old saying: "If you don't know where you're going, any path will get you there."

But if you do know where you're going, it becomes easier to know what path to take.

If my phone rings and somebody says to me, "How do I get to Third and Elm?" well, my first question is going to be, "Where are you right now?"

I've got to know where you are *and* where you want to go.

And then they take action toward it, in a measurable way. This difference between a dream and a goal is *timeline* and *accountability*.

Someday is not a day of the week. You have to check in with yourself or with someone you trust to tell you the truth with no patience for excuses. Someone who will hold you accountable. Excuses are not reasons; they are just excuses. If something is really important, you will do it; if it is not, you will make excuses.

For example, if you don't have a job, then your job is to get a job. You absolutely must work as hard or harder at finding a job as you would at working at an actual job. If you had a job and you would put in fifty hours a week working, then you should put in at least fifty hours a week finding a job. If you had a job and you would be up at 6:30 every day, showered, dressed, and out the door by 7:15, then you should do at least that while *looking* for a job. Posting your name or resume on an online site and then playing video games or watching Netflix all day *is not looking for a job*. Get real with yourself.

You have to identify steps to take toward a measurable outcome. I just gave you some real-world examples.

Third, successful people don't lie to themselves. What I mean is winners deal with the truth as it comes up. They deal with reality. They don't tell themselves, "Oh, this is working out great," when it isn't.

They'll admit when they've hit a dead end and will make a change. They're willing to change direction, but the one thing they're not willing to do is stop. They don't pursue success for a month or a year or two years; they do it *until*. *Until* they succeed. Which is another way of saying that for winners, failure is not an option.

So what does success entail? Taking purposeful action, on a timeline; being honest with yourself, and refusing to quit. Like I said, you are the CEO of YOU, Inc. Since you can't fire you and hire new management, you'd better get right with the boss!

Success Takes Time

In the late 1960s and early 1970s a professor at Stanford University named Walter Mischel wanted to test a question that goes back to the Garden of Eden: How do we resist temptation?[10] In particular, he wanted to understand at what age we begin to be able to control our impulses. He came up with a very simple test. He took a group of children between the ages of four and six and put a marshmallow in front of them, along with a bell. He then would leave the room. They were told that if they rang the bell, he would come back and they could eat the marshmallow. But if they waited for him to come back in fifteen minutes without ringing the bell, they'd get two marshmallows.[11]

You can watch videos of kids trying to resist the temptation of eating that one marshmallow. They squirm. They kick. Some sniff the marshmallow. Some just give up and ring the bell within a minute. The experiment found that children who were able to hold out the longest were the ones who developed creative strategies, like singing songs or covering their eyes and pretending the marshmallow wasn't there.

But then an interesting thing happened. Years later, they checked in on the children who had participated in the experiment, and the ones who held out for the second marshmallow had fewer behavioral problems and higher SAT scores.

This experiment has been rerun a bunch of different ways, and there are all sorts of variables that change the results. (Do the kids trust the person putting the marshmallow out there? Does the amount of time they're asked to wait matter? Do they come from a home where they can trust adults?) But the end result is always that some ability to wait, to delay gratification, is linked to success later on.

And it makes sense. If you can visualize the larger goal that's worth working for (and waiting for), even at a young age, your chances of succeeding in achieving it go up.

Succeed with—Not Off of—Others

As I'm writing this, I'm in the process of shutting down the *Dr. Phil* show as it was known for more than two decades.

I'm not a particularly emotionally expressive person, but shutting down the show gave me the chance to reflect on what it's all been about. Did I stay true to the values that set this whole thing in motion in the first place?

I think back to those first meetings where I had to explain what my show would be, in the absence of Oprah. I summed it up this way: "We're going to talk about things that matter to people who care. We're going to talk about things that aren't much spoken about in polite society, but I'm going to push them to the forefront of American life, in the hopes of saving and improving lives."

My feeling has always been that if responsible people don't talk about impor-

> My feeling has always been that if responsible people don't talk about important problems responsibly, then irresponsible people will talk about important problems irresponsibly.

tant problems responsibly, then irresponsible people will talk about important problems irresponsibly.

One grim example of an issue we took on: 95 percent of people who are molested know the molester. It's got to be one of the most underreported crimes in the country. You have millions of people living in shame their whole lives, letting it ruin their lives. We said we were going to talk about it, and we did.

We kept our promise to deliver commonsense, usable information into people's homes every day for free. We took things that might have required a professional or medical appointment for someone to access, and made them much more accessible.

But I very quickly realized that the "people who care" couldn't just be the audience, it had to be my team as well. There needed to be a sense of mission.

When they submit a show proposal to me, they had to be very clear about the takeaway. If we're going to do a show on parenting children who are behaving like spoiled brats, what are we going to offer that helps the parents and the children? How are they going to be better for having watched this show? How is the viewer better equipped?

It can't be voyeuristic for the sake of voyeurism. If we have a show about a serial killer, it has to have an element on identifying the anti-social behaviors that you might see in your own family or friends, so you can intervene.

Those were my only rules: things that matter, people who care, common sense, usable information. And within that context, the people who work with me got to pitch shows that *they* were passionate about. That's how I came to do shows on fairness in lending, and the pressures that police officers face (a side of the blue line we don't often see).

And that resulted in people on my team going above and beyond, in all kinds of different ways—and building their own consequential knowledge in the process.

I think a lot about the episodes we did with Michelle Knight. She was one of the three women whom Ariel Castro held captive for eleven years. We knew how powerful it would be if she would be willing to tell her story.

So my news producer, Sarah Carden, went to see her. She spent about fifteen days in a row with Michelle Knight. They watched movies together in her hotel room; they went and got their hair done. They built a rapport, and then trust. And thanks to Sarah's work, Michelle told her story on our air with a clarity, directness, and bravery that left me awestruck. Thanks to Sarah's work, she became the first of his three captives to speak out.

You can't pay somebody enough to put in the work Sarah did. They still trade Christmas cards! That's above and beyond. It's passion.

Or I think about Justin Arluck. Justin started as an audience coordinator on the show, basically making minimum wage. He's been promoted at least seven times, and now he's a senior supervising producer.

One of the things I've learned studying success is that you're going to be hard-pressed to find a true sustained success that's a Lone Ranger. Not one time have I seen true success that was obtained by one person, acting on their own. They surrounded themselves with a nucleus of people who wanted them to succeed. They forged relationships with people who wanted them to succeed, and felt like they had a stake in that success. They didn't try to succeed *off* of the sweat or skills of others. They worked to succeed *with* others. They worked to make sure that there were people around them whose consequential knowledge dovetailed with theirs.

It's not enough that I'm passionate. I've searched out and found a group of people who are passionate about the same things I'm passionate about. Different skills, same passion. One of the things I say about my staff is that money is paid, but it's not about the money. You can't pay my producers enough money for the time, the hours, the care, the energy that they put into the stories that they find and pursue, the people they support and deal with, in service of sharing their stories.

So, before we shut down the *Dr. Phil* show in California, I asked a handful of my key people to join me in Texas for my next television project. They have built lives in California. The change will require selling homes, moving families, and uprooting lives. I'm so grateful that, to a person, they all said yes.

Avoid the Envy Trap

All this talk about success is a good reminder that there is a dark side of human nature that I have not spoken about yet. It can be summed up in one word: *envy.*

Envy is the basic part, the ugly part, of human nature that causes people to resent others who have more than they do, or who are happier than they are. It causes people to try to do what in relationship parlance is called "leveling."

There are two ways to level. One way is to puff yourself up, and the other way is to tear another person down. When you can't raise your own ceiling, you lower someone else's floor. And that's like trying to fix your leaky boat by drilling a hole in somebody else's. Envy is not just a sin, as I discuss in the chapter about the decline of religion. It also fuels leveling.

Here's why it's particularly dangerous: because if you want what someone else has, you'll always find someone with more. You will never be satisfied, because envy can't be satisfied. You'll be forever chasing. As I advise people in relationships: "Don't chase the wrong one, because the right one won't run."

The other reason envy is dangerous is that the very thing of which you're envious might not be the truth. You can be envious of someone's carefree financial lifestyle, without realizing they they're on the verge of bankruptcy or deep in debt. You can be envious of someone's perfect-seeming relationship without knowing a thing that goes on behind closed doors. You don't know. You can't know. And so you're envying a social mask. And a social mask, like a real mask, may look good from one perspective, but from another isn't even skin-deep.

Now, I realize saying "don't be envious" doesn't help much. But it's important to recognize that you envy others when you don't feel good about yourself.

The only thing that puts out the fire of envy is self-fulfillment, and self-fulfillment comes, in large part, from consequential knowledge.

POLL RESPONSE

Are you comfortable that you have identified, developed, and continue to develop that skill or talent that puts you in the best position in a competitive marketplace?

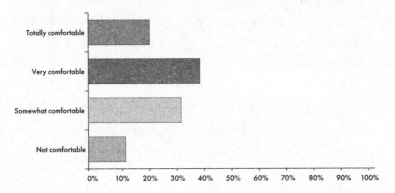

Work Hard to Understand the Way Others See Things

POLL QUESTION

Think back to some meaningful encounters. How good are you at listening and truly understanding the point of view of someone you have a disagreement with?

☐ Very

☐ Somewhat

☐ Not very

☐ Not at all

A couple of years ago, a friend named Frank Luntz invited me to come join a meeting he was holding with some students from the University of Southern California at his home in Los Angeles. He was working with a group of college Democrats and Republicans to try to get them to communicate better. I jumped at the chance and brought a camera crew as well.

Frank is a world-renowned pollster and a communications consultant and just an all-around brilliant guy. He has always had his finger on the pulse of the American people. He's particularly focused on the power of language to move people. Early in his career, he used that skill mainly to the benefit of Republicans. If you've ever heard of Newt Gingrich's Contract with America, or heard someone refer to the "estate tax" as the "death tax" or "energy exploration" instead of "oil drilling," you can thank Frank.

Frank's belief—one that I share—is that words trigger emotional responses. So, when he thinks that an issue is loaded with too much emotion, he tries to calm it down. His point with "energy exploration" is that it is less scary than "oil drilling." By the same token, the "death tax" sounds a lot scarier and more un-American than the estate tax. In fact, it was on his advice that Republicans started using deeply emotional words like *sick*, *corrupt*, and *traitors* to describe Democrats.

For years, Democrats feared his advice—because he helped Republicans outmessage and outmaneuver them.

But in recent years, a couple of things happened to Frank. After the 2012 presidential election, he became deeply upset, not because his side had lost, but because of what he feared was happening to America. As he described it in a magazine article around that time: Americans had become hardheaded, argumentative, and incurious. They didn't want to hear other points of view. They had become tribal and divided in a way that he had never seen before. In his words, "They want to impose their opinions rather than express them." And Frank was disturbed by the role he had played in bringing about this state of affairs.

In 2017, a wildfire in California forced him to evacuate his home. He pledged to use his skills to promote environmental protection, promising to help Democrats as well as Republicans. He didn't change his worldview. He and I still share an abiding belief in capitalism and self-reliance.[1] He and I also share a commitment to calling it like we see it. So, in recent years, he's been blasted by folks like Tucker Carlson for actually looking for common ground on issues like immigration and the environment.[2]

Trying to find common ground is what brought me to Frank's home in late spring 2022, and into a room full of about forty young people who were smart, articulate, and came armed with some pretty strong political views.

At one point, the students were discussing a bill the Florida legislature had passed. It's officially known as HB 1557. In a testament to the power of emotional language, you've probably heard it referred to as the "Don't Say Gay Bill."

The students were having a spirited, but overall respectful and civilized, debate.

In fact, there were some really constructive things going on. One student stopped the debate dead in its tracks by asking, "Who should be making these curriculum decisions?" and several other students tried to come up with an answer. It felt like constructive problem solving. The students seemed to agree that kids needed to learn certain facts of life, but at an age-appropriate time, and in an age-appropriate way. I began to think, "Huzzah, if Congress worked like this, we'd be in a much better place!"

Then one of the students said that what one of his classmates was defending was "like Italian fascism." And the whole tone of the room changed. Frank asked the student if he really wanted to use that term to describe a classmate. The student who had used the term protested, rightly, that he hadn't actually called his classmate a fascist. He had said that the policy being defended was "like fascism." But one of the things Frank has pointed out—and he even wrote a book about this—is that "it's not what you say, it's what people hear." And one student just heard himself called a fascist, and wasn't happy about it.

Another student, who wasn't on one side or the other politically, chimed in to say that what she was watching was "kind of horrifying . . . this doesn't seem to be a politics issue. It seems like you guys just fundamentally don't like each other as people. It seems like this is going beyond your political beliefs and is really an assault on both sides of your characters."

That's when I stepped in to ask the dueling students, "Are you trying to win an argument or are you trying to solve a problem?"

The reply I got from one student was very telling: "We try to win arguments as part of trying to solve a larger problem."

A lot of people think that way. If you can beat your opposition into submission, then you can make some progress. But that's now how things work. As we said in the previous chapter, you can win an argument or you can solve a problem. You can't often do both.

The room was getting tense; the students were dehumanizing each other. They needed to remember there were people behind the beliefs. So I asked them to stand up and pair up, preferably with someone who didn't share their beliefs. It's an exercise I've conducted dozens of times, called a "standing dyad." I had them face each other, a little too close for comfort, in each other's personal space. First I asked them to simply make eye contact, for longer than is normally comfortable. And as they did this, I reminded them that the person in front of them has parents, siblings, they get up in the morning just like you and decide what to wear. They have fears, pride, thoughts, feelings—just like you.

Then I asked each of them to tap the other on the shoulder and say one of four things. I trust you. I don't trust you. I don't know if I trust you. I'd rather not say.

Then I asked each of them to find a new partner and do it again. And then again one more time. And each time, I reminded them: The person across from you is another human being. What have they gone through today? Did they lose a loved one recently? Are they struggling financially? Have they accomplished something they're really proud of?

After the third round, the exercise was done. There was a lot of laughter—some of it relief from being done with the awkwardness, and some of it from the shock of realizing there were unexpected moments of connection.

One of the students volunteered that "there's someone behind these political ideals. Someone dealing with an issue you yourself might be dealing with. It's not all about what we disagree on. . . . I felt very connected. I wasn't even considering their affiliation or their identity. I just saw a human being and had that empathy."

Another student chimed in, "It's a lot harder to say you don't trust someone who you're looking straight at, whereas it's so much easier to hide behind a screen and assume things about people . . . it's a lot different when you're asking me to look at this person and view them as a human being. . . . I realized that I sometimes personally forget to do that."

In fact, more students said they trusted each other in the third round than the second, and more in the second than in the first. Their body language became more open. There was more smiling.

Frank Luntz, who has conducted thousands of focus groups and seen just about everything there is to see about how people interact, was gobsmacked. Shaking his head, he said, "This is a 'holy s—' finding. I want to try this with all of America!" Then he joked that he'd probably get arrested for going around telling people to touch each other.

To me, this isn't so much of a "holy s—" finding as it is a recognition of something we always knew, but forgot as we have retreated to our tribes and behind our screens: if you don't start on a human-to-human basis, then you're building a house on sand.

> **If we don't treat each other as human beings, then all of the various ways in which we can disrespect one another, whether it's crime, violence, mugging, insults, whatever—it all becomes so much easier if you don't regard them personally.**

If we don't treat each other as human beings, then all of the various ways in which we can disrespect one another, whether it's crime, violence, mugging, insults, whatever—it all becomes so much easier if you don't regard them personally.

And if you do regard them personally, then it becomes much harder to disrespect and disregard the worth of that human being. We live in such a fast-paced society that we don't really take time to look at each other and regard each other as human beings.

But taking that time really matters.

Let me give you the most extreme case in which it matters: hostage negotiation.

I've interviewed a number of hostage negotiators over the years, and they'll tell you the best predictor of whether you're going to get hostages out of a situation alive is whether or not the hostage taker believes that you understand why they took them in the first place. That is the number one predictor. And if they believe that you get it, that you understand, whether it's a Muslim thing, whatever the situation, if they believe that you've actually listened, and you get it, you understand why they took them, that's your best shot that they're going to say, "Okay, I've been heard. Somebody gets it. They've listened to me, they understood, so I've made my point."

That's true in a life-or-death situation, and it's just as important in getting someone to agree with you, to at least consider what you have to say, on whatever issue is in front of you. People want to be heard.

You have to understand someone and what makes them tick before you can connect with them. They need to see similarities between you and your values and their own. That's the basis of bonding. And bonding can open the door to progress.

So how do you get there? How do you actively listen? To really understand someone, what is it you need to know? What information will truly tell you who they are?

Well, let's start with what we already know. No, I don't mean pretend to be Sherlock Holmes and say, "Ah, there's a tobacco stain on his finger, so he must smoke . . ." No, there are certain fundamental truths that animate everybody. They're the common characteristics of human functioning.

Write these things on a note card, put it in your wallet or purse, tattoo them on the back of your hand. Before you know anything else about anybody you interact with, you know this:

> The number one fear among all people is rejection.
> The number one need among all people is acceptance.
> If you want to manage, persuade, or convince someone, you have to do it in a way that protects or enhances their self-esteem.
> Everybody—and I mean everybody, including Mother Teresa—approaches every situation with at least some concern about "what's in it for me."
> Everybody—and I mean everybody, not just men out on dates—prefers to talk about things that are important to them personally.
> People hear and incorporate only what they understand.
> People like, trust, and believe those who like them.
> People often do things for reasons that are not immediately apparent.
> Even decent, honorable people can be—and often are— petty and small.
> Everybody—and I mean everybody—wears a social mask. You need to get behind the mask to see the person.

This isn't pessimism. This is realism. And everything in this book is about reconstructing your life on a foundation of what's real.

If that list represents the traits that everyone shares, what questions do you need to ask, what answers do you need in order to understand someone? Here, too, years of experience have yielded what, for me, is a pretty solid list of the Big 7:

1. What do they value and want most in their lives? Are ethics a big deal? Are they defined by money and success? Do they value strength or compassion?
2. What are their expectancies and beliefs about how life does and should work?
3. What resistances or predispositions—fears, biases, prejudices—do they have?
4. What positions or approaches or philosophies are they most likely to accept or reject?
5. What do they need to hear from a person in order to conclude that person is fundamentally "okay" and can be trusted?
6. What sorts of things do they consider relevant?
7. How do they feel about themselves?

Now, these aren't questions that you can just go up and ask someone. It takes time to figure out the answers.

Beyond the "what," you have to get at the "why"—and this is another place where understanding can be lost, or gained.

I tell the people I teach to not only find out what the person across the table wants, but *why*. Everybody has a different kind of currency. As I said earlier, you may find out that what is a level 10 to them is a 2 to you, but also *why* is it *so important* to them. How can it be such a small thing to you and so defining to them? Discovering that answer will be very powerful. Be careful not to assume that you know the answer.

You see it with families all the time. Consider the age-old debate between parents and children on the subject of a curfew. If there's a debate over curfew, I guarantee you that, from the kid's perspective, they want freedom and they think the parents want control.

But in most cases, the parents' "why" is actually different. The parents usually want safety. So the parents are saying that they want their child home because they know that the majority of traffic accidents happen when the bars let out between midnight and 2 a.m.

Once you realize that the parent isn't worried about control, or even the curfew time, then you've opened the door to progress.

What Will It Take to Bring Us Together?

It seems like the last time we were unified as Americans was in the aftermath of the attacks of September 11, 2001. George W. Bush, all of a sudden, became a president for all Americans. He unified us against a common enemy. I don't want us to have to have some horrible disaster or happening to get us singing from the same hymnal again.

Why can't we figure that out without tragedy?

And I'm worried because even tragedies aren't doing the job anymore. There's a terrible rail disaster in Ohio, over 100,000 pounds of toxics substances spill or have to be burned off, fouling the soil, the air, and the water. Within days, one side says, "This happened because liberals don't care about rural America." The other side says, "This happened because conservatives gave in to corporate greed, and this is the result." And the mayor has to come out and say: stop using my people, who have had this terrible thing happen, as political pawns.[3] For a long time, it pissed people off that when something terrible happened, leaders would only offer "thoughts and prayers." Now they don't even offer that—they skip over the thoughts and prayers and go straight to the politics. And too often, we go along with it, allowing people to be turned into pawns, and our fellow Americans into enemies.

When I teach negotiation, I say that when you sit down across from someone, the first thing you say is let's get a list of everything we agree on. If we take the time to invest in that, we may find that our differences are a lot narrower and a lot more manageable. Maybe we see that there's enough commonality to build on.

POLL RESPONSE

Think back to some meaningful encounters. How good are you at listening and truly understanding the point of view of someone you have a disagreement with?

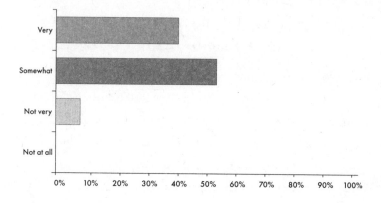

PRINCIPLE #10

Treat Yourself and Others with Dignity and Respect

POLL QUESTIONS

How often do you feel that you are not being treated with dignity and respect?
- ☐ Always
- ☐ Very often
- ☐ Sometimes
- ☐ Never

How often do you consciously treat others with equal or greater dignity than you feel you've been treated with?
- ☐ Always
- ☐ Very often
- ☐ Sometimes
- ☐ Never

Growing up, we all learned the Golden Rule. It shows up several times in the Bible, and in just about every major religion: Do unto others what you would have them do to you. It's a fundamental ethical principle. In fact, you could argue that it is *the* fundamental ethical principle. Everything else is commentary.

That's the idea behind my final rule for societal success: treat yourself and others with dignity and respect.

It's easy to understand, and you've probably heard some version of it all of your life. I'm not trying to reinvent the wheel here, or pretending that this is a mind-bending new insight. I want to refocus all of us on this fundamental principle of coexistence. Coexistence with ourselves, the person we spend the most time with, the person we have to look at in the mirror every day, the person we present as a model to our children.

I start by refocusing on the second half of this rule, "what you would have them do to you." We assume it means that we all want to generally be treated with respect and kindness. But do we? Do we think we deserve those things? Do we treat ourselves that way?

So I want to start with what this means for you personally, because you can't give away what you don't have.

Look, the longest relationship you will have in life is with yourself. Be your own best friend. And because we generate the results in life that we believe we deserve, help yourself generate those results.

If you don't regard yourself with dignity and respect, there's no way you can ever give it to anyone else. Committing to dignity and respect every single day—living it, feeling it, demanding it—will not only change your walk through life; it is necessary to start healing this society one life at a time. It's essential to a healthy and functioning society.

So, what does that commitment require of you? Deep down, or not so deep down, you have to already know that answer. But somehow, some way, we have allowed ourselves to fall below any reasonable standard of logic or common sense when it comes to what we are willing to accept from ourselves or others.

Too many of us have allowed ourselves to be bullied by the Tyranny of the Fringe I've been talking about. I want you to make peace with yourself. I want you to sit down and get out an old-fashioned pen and pad and thoughtfully write down what it is you truly think, feel, and believe about important categories of behaviors, patterns of behavior, events, people, relationships, beliefs, and values in your life.

If you're like me, your first instinct will be to think, "Hey, I can do this in my head while I'm driving to or from work, or walking the dog, or while I'm on the stationary bike or treadmill."

No! You cannot. Trust me when I tell you that it's different when you have to write it down. We function in different modes, and one of the modes is "production mode." Production mode is where you actually have to *actively* crystallize your thoughts enough to put them down in a coherent way, *on paper*. And you can go back and look at your various lists and writings from one day to the next to remind and recommit yourself. But it's there, in black and white, for you to see. As things become clearer in your mind and heart, you can modify what you've written. But you can't just forget it—the way you could if you hadn't written it down.

I highly suggest you get some kind of journal or book you can write in and put a heading at the top of a page, then leave several pages to write on before you put the next heading at the top of a page.

Then, before you start writing under a given heading such as "Values," take some time to really ask yourself some serious questions.

This book, this list, your answers, are for *your eyes only.* You may choose to share some of what you've written with someone later, but it's important to be clear that unless you decide otherwise, no one will see this but you.

That's important because you must, absolutely must, be brutally honest in this private conversation you're about to have with yourself.

Before you write your first word under "Values" you need to construct a timeline. Write down your current page and work backward as far as you can reliably remember and ask yourself, for example, such things as:

> Along the way, what have I consistently placed great importance on? Honesty? Keeping my word? Loyalty? Hard work? Giving my feelings a voice? Controlling my anger? Resisting the temptation to judge others? Being tolerant? Practicing humility? Never giving up on a goal? Speaking up when I feel the need? Again, these are just examples to get you started. The values that are important to you could be any of hundreds of things.

> Have my values changed across time? If so, why did they change? Which ones have changed? Was it a positive change, or did I lower my standards? Did something happen that disrupted my personal compass? What was it? Do I need to deal with that?

> What are my values now, and how are they working for me? Personally? Professionally? Spiritually? Relationally? Familially?

> Can I be proud of the values I embrace today?

> Have I matured or regressed across time?

> Am I in control of my values or have I allowed them to be "hijacked" by giving my power away to others?

It is only when you have done this personal audit concerning your behaviors—including your patterns of behavior, the significant events in your life, the way in which you deal with the people you encounter in your life, the way in which you conduct yourself within the relationships in your life—that you can truly gain a clear view of whether you are treating and conducting yourself with dignity and respect, and therefore whether you are ready to do the same with others in your world too.

I've said many times that I think old sayings get to be old sayings because they are profound; they stand the test of time. The old saying "You should clean your own house first" definitely applies here. Once you have done the work on you, it is time for engaging others more positively, because one thing I know for sure:

You can't give away what you don't have.

But I said treating yourself and others with dignity and respect is about two key ideas:

The first is that you can't give away what you don't have.

The second is that we generate the results in life that we believe we deserve.

If you have been honest and "cleaned your own house," you *know* you deserve "first-class relationships" in which you give and receive treatment defined by dignity and respect.

How often do you see or meet someone who appears to be living a first-class life? Maybe they're in great physical shape. Their hair is trimmed up. They're well groomed. Their clothes, whatever the style, look clean and sharp and pressed. It's clear they've taken some time for themselves. They pull up in a car that's clean. It's not necessarily a fancy car; it just doesn't look like they've eaten their last several meals in it. And when they get out, their shoulders are back and their head is up. They walk forward purposefully, with an air of confidence about them.

There are a lot of people who look at someone like that—maybe you're one of them—and say, "That's for other people, not me. I'm not entitled to that." In fact, a lot of people look at that and start making excuses: "I don't have time to stay fit. I can't afford to get my hair done like that." And again, the story they tell themselves is "That's for those people. That's not for me."

It's not just material goods or individual presentation, because you can be looking at someone from the exact same socioeconomic situation. People deliver that message to themselves in every aspect of life.

A lot of people will see another couple that's out holding hands, or being playful, or laughing or playing a sport or visiting a gallery together, and look at that happiness and joy and they say, "Well, that's for other people. That's not for us."

The only reason someone says something like that is that they don't think they deserve something they want. And if you don't think you deserve that happiness, that fulfillment, that confidence, there is no way you will generate that result in your own life.

As a result, people give up. They give up long before they should. I'm talking about the people who, one day you see them and they're middle-aged, reasonably fit, reasonably active. But then you run into them a couple of years later, and all of a sudden they look like they've aged decades, their walk has become more of a shuffle, and you think, Whoa, what happened?

Meanwhile, you've got my wife, Robin. Back in 2009, she wrote a book called *What's Age Got to Do with It*. She's on the cover, in a form-fitting black outfit, wearing heels (that's about as sophisticated as I'm capable of being when describing the specifics of a woman's outfit), sitting on the number 55, which was her age at the time. The book was a revelation, because *nobody in Hollywood*, especially women, talks about their age. And she put it on the cover of her book. But she did it because she had made a decision that one of the worst things you can do is look at energy, ambition, youthfulness, your desire to learn and to grow—and decide that those things are behind you.

Today, by the way, she still looks *exactly* like she did on the cover of the book. And people look at her and kind of say, must be nice to have that life, like she was born into it. And what they don't know is that she didn't grow up in the life she has now. She made a decision that she *deserved* a big life.

Robin grew up in a small town in Oklahoma. Her father ran a golf driving range, but they didn't have one of those tractors to pick up balls; Robin's job was to grab a bucket and do it by hand. (I joke about how much of a success she could have been if she had worn a helmet.)

She had three older sisters, and her mother made all of their clothes. She got the hand-me-downs. She never wore anything store bought or anything that was made directly for her.

She wanted more, and she created it.

It comes back to something we've already discussed in this book: personal truth. If you believe you're a second-class citizen, then you're going to generate a second-class life.

You're not going to hold yourself to a standard of excellence. You may not reach for that next level of education or that next level of employment. This is very much on my mind right now, because as I write this book, I'm rehabbing from knee surgery. And the physical therapist says that I have to do 75 reps of an exercise—I'm supposed to do 30, and then three sets of 15. And guess what, it hurts like hell! I could cheat and do fewer. I could claim I need to reschedule a rehab session and never quite get around to it—that's a good avoidance tactic. But I grit my teeth and do them. Because I think I deserve to be able to walk effortlessly again. I don't just *want* to be able to play tennis again. I *deserve* it.

> Treating yourself with dignity and respect requires that you stop and say, "What standards do I hold myself to? Do I treat myself in a way that is going to generate for me what I really want?"

Treating yourself with dignity and respect requires that you stop and say, "What standards do I hold myself to? Do I treat myself in a way that is going to generate for me what I really want?"

You've already written down some thoughts about your values. Now, on the foundation of those values, say you're writing a script for what your life would look like in a perfect world. I know there's no perfect world, but let your imagination run wild for a minute. What does your life look like? Do you have what you want in your life? Are you as healthy as you want? Are you as trim as you want? Do you have an exciting job that you want? Do you have interests that you're passionate about? Do you take care of yourself? Do you stand up for yourself? Do you support yourself? Do you believe in yourself? Have you tested your own thoughts and beliefs and values, and feel confident in them?

You need to be able to picture that "perfect world" because that vision tells you who you are and who you want to be. And if you're falling short of that vision, you need to decide what parts of your life you want to keep and what parts you want to change.

That's what I mean when I say that I want you to be who you are on purpose. Don't just be who you are by default; be who you are on purpose.

It's almost impossible to treat yourself with dignity and respect if you're living a life you aren't choosing on purpose.

I can't tell you the number of times I've sat across from a patient in my office or a guest on my show and said some version of "You have my full attention here. We're not leaving until we come up with a solution to your problem. We're going to take action; we're going to use verbs. We're going to get you whatever you need—a therapist, a trainer, a lawyer—whatever you need to put your life on a different track. My question for you is 'Do you feel worthy of the attention you're getting and the support I'm offering?'"

Almost invariably, they'll start crying, because they don't feel worthy.

It's as if they're saying, "I don't feel worthy of being chosen out of the tens of thousands of letters I know you get. I don't feel worthy of you sitting here, making eye contact with me, focusing on my entire life and offering me all this help. I don't know why you're doing it and I don't feel worthy of this."

Instead of coddling them, I'll say, "Well, maybe you're not. You know yourself better than I do, and, knowing yourself, if you know you're not worthy of this, then maybe I'm wasting my time. You've got to claim it. You've got to claim the right to have this help and embrace it or I'm wasting my time."

I work with them until they say, "Okay, I claim this. It's my moment. It's my time. It's my turn, and I claim it, right here, right now. I do it for me and I do it for my family."

Claiming it. That's the first step in generating the results in life you believe you deserve. Then, and only then, can you treat other people the same way. Hence, you can't give away what you don't have. You can't give away dignity you don't have. You can't give away respect you haven't earned.

But once you have those things, you're powerful. And you can have a powerful, positive effect. Some people feel they're at their strongest when they're angry. "You get me angry, by God, I'll be something to contend with!" In reality, that's when you're the weakest because you're angry when you feel violated. And if you're violated, that means you've been victimized. And being a victim is weak.

What you want to do is say, "We have a situation here that needs handling. And I am a problem manager, so I am going to go in and handle this because I am worthy of a different outcome. I don't need to be angry, I don't need to be hysterical, I don't need to be accusatory, I just need to be focused."

You're at your strongest when you don't need to feel angry toward others. You're at your strongest when you can be generous with the dignity and respect and grace that you've earned.

I've always said that I don't have to love everything about someone to love them. I don't have to love everything about somebody to get along with them. And I always tell people that when you're arguing or have a disagreement, your goal shouldn't be to win. The goal should be a statement like "I want you to hear me, and you don't even necessarily need to respond, I just want you to hear me. I just want to know that you've heard me and you understand my point of view. And then across time, I hope we'll find a way to common ground enough of the time. But you don't need to agree with me. My goal is not for you to agree with my point, just that you hear me. And I want to do the same thing with you: I want to hear you. And don't ask me to agree or disagree, just let's hear each other, and then we'll take a step back and think about it."

No disagreement provides license to be entitled, disrespectful, and disloyal. And I do mean disloyal. We have a duty to be loyal Americans. To be loyal to each other.

It's one of the reasons I'm so disturbed by the fact that 2021 was the worst year on record for bad behavior by people on airplanes. So the Federal Aviation Administration put in place a zero-tolerance policy, and 2022 . . . was even worse. Verbal abuse, physical abuse, noncompliance, intoxication—all of them up.[1] To me, in the same way that a jury is a microcosm of society, an airplane is a microcosm of community—it's a test of how we get through a not-always-enjoyable, not-always-predictable experience together. Most of the time, we do okay. We get along. We follow the rules; we tolerate the screaming child. But it seems like recently we look for conflict before commonality, confrontation instead of cooperation.

That's one of the reasons I was both fascinated and disgusted during the 2023 State of the Union address when Representative Marjorie Taylor Greene yelled "Liar!" at President Biden. In that moment, she debased herself, Congress, and our country. She didn't treat herself or anyone else with dignity and respect.

Something is deeply, deeply wrong with an American who has been elected to Congress yelling "liar" at America's president. It is just plain wrong. This is not the mores and folkways of our government or our society. What I saw was an erosion of values. And an erosion of character.

I want to be clear, I'm no great fan of Joe Biden, and I've called him out earlier in this book. But if I had him on the show, or met him on the street, or attended an event he was at—I would treat him with dignity and respect for no other reason than that he occupies the office. I would show him respect for what he did in getting to the office. And I would try to find things we do agree on.

We all need to ask ourselves: What message have I sent, as a citizen, as a voter, that we've elected people who think it's okay to behave that way? What can I do to demand and provide dignity and respect?

Because believe it or not, I think we can solve a lot with civility.

POLL RESPONSES

How often do you feel that you are not being treated with dignity and respect?

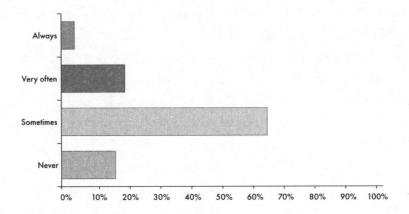

How often do you consciously treat others with equal or greater dignity than you feel you've been treated with?

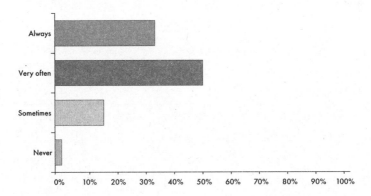

I ask the second question in particular, because if we are going to stop the cycle of confrontation and disrespect, we need to be treating people *better* than we feel we've been treated. It's the only way to stop the slide.

Step onto the Number Line

One of my favorite teaching tools, although I've only used it four or five times over twenty years, is a long, plastic ruler that rolls out on the floor. It's a foot wide, about thirty feet long, and it's marked with really big numbers—zero to 83.

Those aren't markings of distance. They're markings of age. Eighty-three years is, more or less, our average life expectancy, a bit less for men and a bit more for women.

It's a simple visual to see a timeline of your life stretched out in front of you, right? But I promise you, every time I use it, it's amazingly effective in getting people to focus on the most basic reality of life: that it's finite.

I roll it out and ask the person I am focused on to step onto the life ruler at zero and walk along until they reach their age. If they are 62, they walk past 20, 30, 40, and 50 years until stopping on their age, 62 years.

They inevitably look over their shoulder and see how much of their life is over, gone, behind them. By contrast, there's not a ton of space representing how much of their life is left, staring them in the face. That future that once seemed so endless, that horizon that once seemed so distant, isn't. A whole lot behind, and the harsh reality, not much ahead. For this 62-year-old, about 75 percent of their life is over, and 25 percent lies ahead.

It makes you realize that getting up today and doing what you do, not because it is what you want to do, but simply because it is what you did yesterday, is just not okay anymore. It will only succeed in doing one thing for you, and that is getting you to the end of that ruler.

It makes you realize that putting up with the BS you put up with, not because you want to, not because it makes any sense, but simply because it is what you put up with yesterday, is just not okay anymore. Again, it will only succeed in pushing you along toward the end of that ruler.

Doing and putting up with certain things *you did not choose for your life* might move you down the number line, but it doesn't move you *forward*. Days turn into weeks, weeks turn into months, months turn into years, and you look over your shoulder and the only life you will ever have has fast slipped away.

The questions become obvious:

> What do you want to do with the rest of your life?
>
> How do you want to spend it?
>
> With whom and focused on what?
>
> How do you want to feel?

When you get to the inevitable end, do you want to look back and say, "I lived those final years of my life"—whether that be five, fifteen, or twenty-five years—"with the courage of my authentic convictions"? Or, "Did I let someone *assign me* a position so I didn't make waves for others? Was I true to myself, or did I get intimidated and become invisible?"

I'll be transparent here and tell you I have personally done this exercise.

One day, several years back, I stood in my television studio on the world-famous Paramount lot in Hollywood. Shooting was done for the day. The studio was empty. The bright lights were off; the cameras had canvas hoods over them. The stage was lit dimly by an overhead night-light. Maybe it's because a television studio is built for the hustle and bustle of a production—the excited, energetic audience, the producers running around, the crew moving cameras and chairs and furniture around the set—that when it's quiet, it feels *extra* quiet. This night, it was just me and my dog Maggie, an amazing rescue I had had since she was eight weeks old and who was my faithful sidekick for thirteen years. She was supposedly a Lab-husky mix but turned out to be a purebred Korean Jindo. More importantly she was my constant companion who devoted her entire existence to protecting me and staying by my side.

I intended to spend a few quiet moments on the set alone, reflecting on what had transpired that day. I was just kind of looking around, taking it all in, when I noticed the life ruler, rolled up tightly on the right edge of the stage, ready to be used with a guest the next morning. I anchored the end with my foot and unrolled it with a push. I slowly, methodically walked to my age. If someone walked in at that moment, they might have thought I was on a tightrope.

Upon arrival at my age, a number I had celebrated with my family just a few months earlier, I reflexively looked over my shoulder. I was startled how much was behind me and how so very little was left in front of me. I actually said it out loud, "So . . . whatcha gonna do, big boy, Dr. Common Sense? Whatcha gonna do?"

I sat on the edge of the stage with Maggie. She had a habit of lying right up against me. She would always put one paw on my leg and used it as a motion detector so if she fell asleep and I moved, she wouldn't miss it and fall behind!

"Whatcha gonna do?"

I actually answered the question, but I did so in two ways.

I answered what I wanted to do with the rest of my life.

But I also answered with as much, if not more, passion and resolve about what I absolutely would *not* allow to be part of the rest of my life.

I started this book by telling you that I'd ask you to write some things down and make some observations and commitments as we went along. Now, as we reach the end, I want you to do that one more time. Before you answer, realize that you are talking about a finite, absolutely limited time left in this life. I don't want you to get to the end and say, "I had a chance, I got a wake-up call and I didn't do anything about it. I just kept riding along wherever the river took me."

What do you want to do with the rest of your life?

What will you *not* allow to be a part of the rest of your life?

No amount of guilt can solve the past, and no amount of anxiety can change the future. But actions can.

So, I think the answers will be as many and varied as the people giving them. Some of you have told me over the years that you aren't sure where to start in articulating such broad and important life decisions.

A few of my own examples might stimulate your thinking.

On the "what I *want to do* with my time left in this world" part of the equation, I began by listing what was really, truly important to me. I gave myself permission to not worry, just for the purposes of this exercise, about being selfish. I want you to give yourself the same permission.

Predictably, high on my list is taking care of and sharing time with the people in my life whom I deeply care about. Also high on my list: spending my time doing things that matter, *really* matter in this world. For me, this means "being of service." It's why, in the midst of a busy life, I find myself flying all over the country to do what I can to draw attention to the cause of people who I believe have been wrongly convicted of crimes. Frankly, being of service, which feels really important to me now, was not on my short list when I was back in my teens and early twenties. Proof that we do grow and evolve, I suppose. Back then it was more about survival. I don't share this to make myself look good or to "virtue signal." What I consider being of service you may not even value or may even consider to be a negative. The point is, I don't care what anyone else thinks. It matters to *me*. I believe in it and that's what counts when you decide how to use your time.

For me, when I really looked inside for answers, it was about more than my golf score, or a well-manicured lawn. (Which is good because I'm a crummy golfer and have never owned a lawn mower.) We have all seen the T-shirt with the words "He who dies with the most toys wins!" Funny; I get the joke, but it is just that—a joke. It isn't even almost true.

Another item on my list: I wanted to be able to look back and have the peace of mind that comes from knowing that I had done everything I could to ensure that those I loved would be safe and secure in their lives when I am no longer around to help make it so. I don't mean to insult any of them by suggesting that they wouldn't survive without me. In fact, they're all quite competent in every aspect of life. But, as I said, give yourself permission to be selfish for the purposes of this exercise. For this window of time, it is about you and what you want to do with the rest of your life; what is important to *you*, not someone else.

It was my last priority where I felt some friction, some unfinished business. I was feeling unsettled as Maggie and I sat there on the edge of the stage. I swear to you that dog was an absolute empath. If something unsettled me, she sensed it, made eye contact with me, and never looked away until whatever was amiss got resolved. She went on alert.

As I sat there, I knew I had provided well for my family. I knew our boys would be taken care of, although, thankfully, they have both been hugely successful in their own right. My wife, Robin, our sons, and our grandchildren would be okay financially. I also knew they are all mentally, emotionally, socially, and physically healthy and thriving, a blessing I can only pray will continue. They all get along beautifully and it is comforting to know they have each other. As the saying goes, you have your first child for you, but you have your second child for the first.

Robin and I also raised our boys in a spiritually rich environment. For my part, I taught them they could come to me with anything, not just for the help and counsel I could offer in this life, but because I knew it was great practice for getting comfortable going to their Heavenly Father. That way, I knew they would never be alone.

I also knew they would take care of their mother, just as she had taken care of them. On its face, it seems like: check, check, check. All the boxes were checked. Wherever in God's plan that number line would be finished for me, I wouldn't have unfinished business.

But Maggie wasn't buying it!

What was bothering me so much?

I began to have an inkling then, and it became much, much clearer to me as each year passed. It's everything I've been writing about in this entire book. I could influence things in our family. I could make sure that they would be okay financially, spiritually, mentally, and emotionally. I could help make sure they were socially well-adjusted and passionately engaged in their lives.

But what about the country they were going to have to do it all in? What about the country they were going to live in and raise their children in? That was the box I couldn't check. Short of a cult or a compound, you can't live your life walled off from the world, untouched by the reality around you.

I was unsettled by the troubling trends, cracks in the foundation of who we are as individuals, families, a society, and a nation.

I saw the beginnings of this Tyranny of the Fringe I have been writing about.

I was concerned with the questions, erosion of values we've wrestled with throughout this book.

What has happened to common sense?

What has happened to timeworn values?

What has happened to accountability and hard work as guideposts for living?

What has happened to respect for demonstrable truth and freedom of speech and thought?

What has happened to the family unit so critical to the success of this country?

What has happened to the rule of law?

What has happened that caused us to start to reward bad behavior in America?

What has happened that has handed control of the narrative to the loudest voice?

What has happened to cause us to be so intimidated that we are willing to remain quiet just so others remain comfortable and don't have to answer legitimate questions?

What has happened that has focused us more on winning arguments than solving problems?

That's why I could not find peace.

Too many unanswered questions. That was the tension in me that Maggie was sensing.

I think, in many ways, I started to write this book that day sitting there with Maggie on that dimly lit stage.

How about you?

Do any of those concerns block you from living the rest of your life with peace and confidence in your heart, the way you really want?

I said I personally answered the question of how I wanted to spend the rest of my life in two ways. One was a description of what I wanted to achieve. The second was what I absolutely did not want to spend the rest of my life experiencing. What I did not want to allow to take up *any* of the time I had left, however much time that may be.

I knew in that moment that I did not want to get to the end of my life and look back and regret having allowed others to dictate what I did, or to have people taking up my time if I did not want them taking up my time, time I did not want to invest in them or allow them to absorb. I knew in that moment that I did not want people in my space if, while they were there, in my head I was secretly screaming, "Will you just shut up and go away!"

I knew I did not want to be around people who visit negativity upon me, people who, for whatever reason, I just did not want to be part of my life. I knew in a nanosecond that I did not want to spend one minute of the rest of my life with people who try to control me, bully me, manipulate me, guilt me, or use me as a vehicle to draw attention to things I don't believe in or endorse.

That meant I had to perfect a very specific skill and develop or, more accurately, refine a very important trait.

The skill I had to perfect was learning 101 Ways to Say "NO!"

NO, I do not want you to come over and tell me about something I'm not interested in investing time and energy into.

NO, I'm not believing your story about why you are a victim.

NO, I'm not abandoning everything I don't just *believe* but *know* to be true just because it is making headlines or trending on X (formerly known as Twitter). Up is up and down is down and, NO, you can't will that to be different.

NO, I won't blindly let you begin to steer my family with some theory important to you but with no basis in fact or history.

NO, I won't support some plan you have for reaping benefits without expending effort. NO free ride.

NO, I won't listen to you judge me for not complying. You can call me an SOB, but you are going to do it long-distance.

NO, I won't allow you to use my name to further your bizarre project that you are pursuing instead of getting a job.

NO, I won't stop speaking the truth because people threaten to "cancel" me for asking empirically based questions.

NO, I won't tell you what you want to hear so you won't get upset and assassinate my character.

And, NO, I won't change my mind because you are offended. I know what I know, I have the science to prove it, and you haven't shown me one shred of evidence to the contrary.

In retrospect, I have always felt this way. Events of late have just deepened my resolve and caused me to hone the skill.

The trait I had to refine actually seems contradictory in that I spend so much of my life working to patiently meet people where *they are* while at the same time urgently, relentlessly petitioning for change. Change of mind, heart and spirit. Calling on people to be who they are on purpose.

But saying "no" and pushing for change are in service of the same goal—getting us back on track.

And to do that, we don't need to leap tall buildings in a single bound. Even small steps, especially when made by a significant number of people, can alter the collective personality of America and put this amazing country back on track much faster than you could ever imagine.

You can change your trajectory. You make a "life decision" and then you live it every day. Start being who you are on purpose, because someday soon, if you're not there already, there's going to be less number line ahead of you than behind you—more yesterdays than tomorrows.

And start paying attention to how your actions impact the people around you, whether what you're doing is getting you the outcome that you want or not.

———

I'll conclude where I began, with optimism.

At my age, I've spent quite a few years as an adult living in a country that I thought was fairly predictable. The values, whether we adhered to them or not, were fairly well-known in terms of right and wrong, mores and folkways. We had clear guideposts, and we may not have liked them all but we certainly knew what they were. It all served to keep us up on the highway. We didn't veer off into ditches all that often.

We always had people who would come up with weird ideas and conspiracy theorists who tried to get people to ignore the messy truth. More or less, though, everybody knew where the guardrails were and we stayed within them.

What I've seen happen in recent years is that we've had our narrative hijacked, our map rewritten, and it's caused an erosion of confidence, an erosion of values, and it's caused our collective personality to have a confidence crisis. We're questioning a lot of things about ourselves—and it's *good* to question things about yourself—but we're often questioning the wrong things, the very things that have made this country a great place to live and a beacon of freedom and hope to the world.

We've almost begun to believe the loud accusers: that every white person is a racist, for example. Or that anyone who has a concern about how we're handling gender identity in young people is a hateful transphobe, or that every gun owner is an advocate of violence. It feels like everybody is accusing somebody of something and nobody is focusing on what we all share.

It's part of why seven out of every ten Americans feel our country is on the wrong track, and have felt that way for over a year—that's the largest, longest sustained bout of national pessimism on record.[1]

But here's where the optimism comes in. We've always been in situations where we have had differences. And as I wrote earlier, when

I'm in a negotiation, the first thing I say is "Okay, first let's focus on what we agree on. Let's get a list of all the things that we agree on because if we'll do that, we may find that what we disagree on is a lot less than we thought going in."

Right now, the people who are spreading divisiveness are effectively saying, "My narrow agenda, which is everything to me, has to be everything to you in order for us to get along."

But here are two more reasons for optimism.

First, the loudest voices aren't necessarily the most numerous voices. We're talking about very small segments of society dominating our societal conversation. And we're going to get them back into proportion.

Second, with this book, you now have the awareness, the tools, the tactics, and the strategies to do just that. You have the ability to say, "I hear you, and I see you. But I also need you to understand that you're being selfish about this. I understand this is everything to you. And I'm willing to find a way for us to coexist, with mutual respect at best, and mutual tolerance at worst. But I will not listen to you simply because you are the loudest voice. I will not allow you to bully me, threaten me, coerce me, or cancel me into abandoning what I believe. I will not allow you to substitute intent for evidence of effectiveness. I can coexist with you, but that doesn't mean I'm going to start disavowing everything I think, feel, and believe in order to get along with you."

For a long time, it has felt like there's nothing to put us together and nothing to bind us together.

That's what I hope this book has provided you—an expression of the values that form the foundation of our great country; principles that allow you, as an individual, to be who you are on purpose and, in the process, to begin acting in ways that will bind us together as a nation. It's time to trade complaint for collaboration and anger for progress.

Together, let's define a new day.

Acknowledgments

There's an old saying: when you see a turtle on a fence post, you know he didn't get up there by himself. There's not much in life I've achieved on my own, and this book is no exception. So, some thank-yous are in order.

That starts with my wife, Robin, who is my partner in all things. Robin has always encouraged me not to confuse success with passion and has reminded me that true success comes from the pursuit of passion. And, of course, it was Robin who reminded me sitting together at the island in our kitchen that I have more to do and more to offer. She specifically said I had a duty to bring some common sense to a world that seemed to have forgotten how, when, and where to use it. This book is a result of that reminder.

I'm very grateful to Bill Dawson, who has been a decades-long friend, confidant, advisor, supporter, critic, researcher, and rewriter. He's a great—and I mean great—trial lawyer with whom I worked on many trials in years past. Bill constantly pushed me to make "my case" stronger and immerse myself in the facts supporting all sides of an issue. It is such a blessing to have Bill as my trusted, elder "go-to." He makes me better and made this book better.

In "prosecuting" my arguments, Bill was joined by Jeff Nussbaum, who served as a spirited intellectual and ideological sparring partner. Absolutely invaluable.

I talked in this book about my "brain room" of crackerjack researchers, so let me pull back the curtain on who they are: Barbara Laubenthal, Kyra Davidson, and Krystal Colon. They are the team that has made sure that this book is empirically and evidence-based. If there's a factual error or misstated conclusion in here, you can bet that's on me, not them.

Lisa Clark, who has helped shepherd so many of my projects, provided invaluable help on everything ranging from creating the "brain room" to sharpening content to organization in the hectic final stages.

I'm grateful to everyone whom you see referenced in this book for offering me their time, perspective, and insight—and allowing me to offer their insights to you.

Jonathan Karp immediately caught the vision and mission of this book. Thank you and Jennifer Long for your invaluable insight along the way. I am excited to be publishing again with Simon & Schuster. Thank you too to Paul Choix for your editorial expertise. Thanks to Jan Miller and Shannon Miser-Marven, my literary agents, partners, and friends for over twenty years. They do so much more than it is reasonable to expect, and bring to their work such passion and commitment to the content and the end product.

I also need to thank my sons Jay and Jordan, who were the initial inspiration for me doing this book. As I watched Jay and Erica and Jordan and Morgan doing such a great job raising their children, I realized how much work we all have to do to give my grandchildren—and all of our children—a better America and better world in which they can flourish.

Perhaps most importantly, I want to thank the millions and millions of viewers who have been on this journey with me over the last twenty-five years. Thank you for teaching me so much and trusting me enough to share your lives' challenges, setbacks, and triumphs. I've never taken you for granted, and I never will.

Lastly, so much of what I learned in life I have learned from the competition of athletics, both college football and tennis. I want to thank all the coaches who pushed me. They taught me that you don't celebrate losses; not everybody gets a trophy. So much of my life was shaped by a simple lesson of competition: if you want better you need to do better. When you're down you are not out as long as you don't stop trying. Somehow you just might find a way to win because you didn't give up; that truly has proven to translate to life.

So, thank you to all of those coaches who didn't accept any of my excuses. I'm endlessly blessed to have the opportunity to impart that same lesson.

Notes

Introduction: We've Got Issues

1 *Whether you think they should or shouldn't:* Bill Hussar et al., "Reading Performance," in *The Condition of Education 2020*, NCES 2020-144, US Department of Education (Washington, DC: National Center for Education Statistics, 2020), https://nces.ed.gov/pubsearch/pubsinfo. asp?pubid=2020144.

2 *The US Department of Education and Literacy Inc.:* "About Us," Literacy Inc., n.d., https://literacyinc.com/.

3 *More than half of Americans:* Siena, "84% Say Americans Being Afraid to Exercise Freedom of Speech Is a Serious Problem," Siena College Research Institute, March 21, 2022, ƒhttps://scri.siena.edu/2022/03/21/84-say-americans-being-afraid-to-exercisefreedom-of-speech-is-a-serious-problem/.

4 *Stanford Law School's dean for diversity, equity, and inclusion:* George Will, "Expensively Credentialed, Negligibly Educated Stanford Brats Threw a Tantrum," *Cullman Times*, March 16, 2023, https://www.cullmantimes.com/george-will-expensively-credentialed-negligibly-educated-stanford-brats-threw-a-tantrum/article_9c164b6c-c34c-11ed-a4e8-aba061e7fb11.html.

5 *"If you're not overtly one of 'us'":* Tess Winston, "With Some of My Fellow Stanford Law Students, There's No Room for Argument," *Washington Post*, April 3, 2023, https://www.washingtonpost.com/opinions/2023/04/03/stanford-law-school-intimidation-of-moderates/.

6 *Several judges have already announced:* James Gordon, "Federal Judges Announce They Will Refuse to Hire Clerks from Stanford Law School after Woke Students and Diversity Dean Ambushed Conservative Member of the Bench: 'They Terrorize People into Submission and Self-

Censorship,'" *Daily Mail*, April 2, 2023, https://www.dailymail.co.uk /news/article-11929519/Federal-judges-announce-refuse-hire-clerks-Stan ford-Law-School-woke-students.html?ito=email_share_article-top.

Chapter 1: The Price and Consequences of Disruption

1 *Yet would it surprise you to learn:* Megan Trimble, "U.S. Kids More Likely to Die Than Kids in 19 Other Nations," *U.S. News & World Report*, January 11, 2018, https://www.usnews.com/news/best-countries/articles/2018-01-11/us -has-highest-child-mortality-rate-of-20-rich-countries.

2 *Two hundred and seventy-seven lives:* Jesse C. Baumgartner, Evan D. Gumas, and Munira Z. Gunja, "Too Many Lives Lost: Comparing Overdose Mortality Rates and Policy Solutions Across High-Income Countries," blog, Commonwealth Fund, May 19, 2022, https://doi.org/10.26099/r689-fk36.

3 *we've dropped to twenty-seventh:* Susan Rotermund et al., "Executive Summary: Elementary and Secondary STEM Education," Science and Engineering Indicators, July 8, 2021, https://ncses.nsf.gov/pubs/nsb20211.

4 *45 million Americans are functionally illiterate:* "Literacy Statistics," National Literacy Institute, n.d., https://www.thenationalliteracyinstitute.com/literacy -statistics.

5 *But with postmodernism, it's all about ideology:* Daniel Palmer, "Explainer: What Is Postmodernism?" The Conversation, January 2, 2014, http://the conversation.com/explainer-what-is-postmodernism-20791.

6 *It's a form of "self-referential" thinking:* Christopher Butler, *Postmodernism: A Very Short Introduction* (Oxford: Oxford University Press, 2003).

7 *In* this context *that's what I'm talking about:* Sheelah Kolhatkar, "The C.E.O. of Anti-Woke, Inc.," *New Yorker*, December 12, 2022, https://www.new yorker.com/magazine/2022/12/19/the-ceo-of-anti-woke-inc.

8 *The term was used several times:* Tonya Mosley and Serena McMahon, "Made Famous by Nixon, the Phrase 'Silent Majority' Resurfaces for Trump's 2020 Reelection," WBUR, July 23, 2020, https://www.wbur.org/hereandnow /2020/07/23/what-is-silent-majority-trump-nixon.

9 *Some people feel that publicly:* Aja Romano, "Why We Can't Stop Fighting about Cancel Culture," Vox, December 30, 2019, https://www.vox.com /culture/2019/12/30/20879720/what-is-cancel-culture-explained-history -debate.

10 *Last year, for the first time, church membership:* Jeffrey Jones, "U.S. Church Membership Falls Below Majority for First Time," Gallup, March 29, 2021, https://news.gallup.com/poll/341963/church-membership-falls-below -majority-first-time.aspx.

PART ONE: AMERICA'S DAILY FOCUS HAS CHANGED

Chapter 2: Think Freely, Speak Freely

1 *A study conducted in 2019:* Alexander Ritter et al., "How Words Impact on Pain," *Brain and Behavior* 9, no. 9 (August 1, 2019), https://doi.org/10.1002/brb3.1377.

2 *And of course, I've spoken to countless patients:* Ann Pietrangelo, "Effects of Emotional Abuse: Short and Long-Term, PTSD, Recovery," Healthline, May 16, 2018, https://www.healthline.com/health/mental-health/effects-of-emotional-abuse.

3 *For some of us, when we redirect our minds:* Christopher N. Cascio et al., "Self-Affirmation Activates Brain Systems Associated with Self-Related Processing and Reward and Is Reinforced by Future Orientation," *Social Cognitive and Affective Neuroscience* 11, no. 4 (April 2016): 621–29, https://doi.org/10.1093/scan/nsv136.

4 *But for people with low self-esteem to begin with:* Dr. Peggy DeLong, "When Positive Affirmations Don't Work: What You Can Do Instead," July 11, 2021, https://drpeggydelong.com/when-positive-affirmations-dont-work-what-you-can-do-instead/.

5 *A prime example occurred at Oberlin:* Jeannie Suk Gersen, "What If Trigger Warnings Don't Work?" *New Yorker*, September 28, 2021, https://www.newyorker.com/news/our-columnists/what-if-trigger-warnings-dont-work.

6 *As a result, we ended up with:* Gersen.

7 *One philosophy professor at Cornell:* Kate Manne, "Why I Use Trigger Warnings," *New York Times*, September 19, 2015, https://www.nytimes.com/2015/09/20/opinion/sunday/why-i-use-trigger-warnings.html.

8 *Doctors have come to realize:* "Living with Germs Has Its Upside. Don't Overdo Cleanliness," *The Science of Health* (blog), University Hospitals, April 12, 2022, https://www.uhhospitals.org/blog/articles/2022/04/living-with-germs-has-its-upside.

9 *What's more, the resolution said:* Michael T. Nietzel, "Cornell University Rejects Students' Call for Trigger Warnings," *Forbes*, April 6, 2023, https://www.forbes.com/sites/michaeltnietzel/2023/04/06/cornell-university-rejects-students-call-for-trigger-warnings/.

Chapter 3: "Inclusive Language" Isn't Inclusive, and It's Barely Language

1 *Heaven forbid you refer to the room:* Leah Asmelah, "Texas Realtor Group Says It Will No Longer Use the Word 'Master' to Describe Bedrooms and Bathrooms in Its Listings," CNN, June 25, 2020, https://www.cnn.com/2020/06/25/us/master-houston-association-of-realtors-trnd/index.html.

2 *Heck, you're not even supposed to say "American":* Nick Mordowanec, "Stanford Slammed for Putting 'American' on Forbidden Word List: 'Take That,'" *Newsweek,* December 20, 2022, https://www.newsweek.com/stanford-criticism-slammed-putting-american-forbidden-word-language-list-1768543.

3 *In this guide, the university's Information Technology:* "IT Inclusive Language Guide," *University of Washington IT Connect* (blog), April 12, 2023, https://itconnect.uw.edu/guides-by-topic/identity-diversity-inclusion/inclusive-language-guide/.

4 *Do the French feel insulted:* Kevin Rawlinson, "AP Apologises and Deletes Widely Mocked Tweet about 'the French,'" *Guardian,* January 28, 2023, https://www.theguardian.com/media/2023/jan/28/ap-issues-clarification-over-its-advice-not-to-use-term-the-french.

5 *A poll done of people of Latin American descent:* Luis Noe-Bistamante, Lauren Mora, and Mark Hugo Lopez, "About One-in-Four U.S. Hispanics Have Heard of Latinx, but Just 3% Use It," Pew Research Center, August 11, 2020, https://www.pewresearch.org/hispanic/2020/08/11/about-one-in-four-u-s-hispanics-have-heard-of-latinx-but-just-3-use-it/.

6 *Another poll found that 40 percent of Latinos:* Luisita Lopez Torregrossa, "Many Latinos Say 'Latinx' Offends or Bothers Them. Here's Why," NBC News, December 14, 2021, https://www.nbcnews.com/think/opinion/many-latinos-say-latinx-offends-or-bothers-them-here-s-ncna1285916.

7 *And by the way, the exact same thing:* Meera E. Deo, "Why BIPOC Fails," *Virginia Law Review* 107, no. 115 (June 6, 2021), https://virginialawreview.org/articles/why-bipoc-fails/.

8 *Sounds pretty inclusive, except white Democrats:* Amy Harmon, "BIPOC or POC? Equity or Equality? The Debate Over Language on the Left," *New York Times,* November 1, 2021, sec. U.S., https://www.nytimes.com/2021/11/01/us/terminology-language-politics.html.

9 *Suggested alternatives:* "Homeless," Diversity Style Guide, February 20, 2021, https://www.diversitystyleguide.com/glossary/homeless-homelessness/; APStylebook [@APStylebook], "New in AP Style: Homeless Is Generally Acceptable as an Adjective to Describe People without a Fixed Residence. Avoid the Term 'the Homeless.' Instead: Homeless People, People without

Housing or People without Homes. Mention That a Person Is Homeless Only When Relevant," tweet, Twitter, May 28, 2020, https://twitter.com/APStylebook/status/1266057234213220352.

10 *And it gets even more ridiculous:* Nicholas Kristof, "Inclusive or Alienating? The Language Wars Go On," *New York Times*, February 1, 2023, https://www.nytimes.com/2023/02/01/opinion/inclusive-language-vocabulary.html.

11 *The American Medical Association:* American Medical Association and Association of American Medical Colleges, "Advancing Health Equity: A Guide to Language, Narrative and Concepts," 2021, https://www.ama-assn.org/system/files/ama-aamc-equity-guide.pdf.

12 *But as the journalist George Packer:* George Packer, "The Moral Case Against Equity Language," *Atlantic*, March 2, 2023, https://www.theatlantic.com/magazine/archive/2023/04/equity-language-guides-sierra-club-banned-words/673085/.

13 *For example, the San Francisco Board of Supervisors:* Phil Matier, "SF Board of Supervisors Sanitizes Language of Criminal Justice System," *San Francisco Chronicle*, August 11, 2019, https://www.sfchronicle.com/bayarea/philmatier/article/SF-Board-of-Supervisors-sanitizes-language-of-14292255.php.

14 *What I do know is that Marshall:* "Justice Marshall, on 'Afro-American': Yes," *New York Times*, October 17, 1989, https://www.nytimes.com/1989/10/17/us/justice-marshall-on-afro-american-yes.html.

15 *However, hate speech that threatens:* David Hudson, "Is Hate Speech Protected by the First Amendment?" Foundation for Individual Rights and Expression, February 8, 2022, https://www.thefire.org/news/hate-speech-protected-first-amendment.

16 *As I write this, a bill was passed by the Michigan House:* Timothy Nerozzi, "Michigan House Passes Bill Making Wrong Pronouns a Felony, Fineable Up to $10,000," Yahoo News, June 30, 2023, https://news.yahoo.com/michigan-house-passes-bill-making-144541245.html.

Chapter 4: It's the 2020s, but We're Living in *1984*

1 *But one thing most serious analysts:* David McRae, "The Inflation Reduction Act Will Not Reduce Inflation," State Treasury of Mississippi, 2020, https://treasury.ms.gov/2022/08/19/mcrae-the-inflation-reduction-act-will-not-reduce-inflation/.

2 *Democrats* and *Republicans in Congress came together:* Patrick T. McHenry [R-NC-10], "H.R.3746—118th Congress (2023-2024): Fiscal Responsibility Act of 2023," June 3, 2023, 2023-05-29, http://www.congress.gov/bill/118th-congress/house-bill/3746.

3 *Look at how we have reframed an obesity epidemic:* "Childhood Obesity Facts," Overweight and Obesity, Centers for Disease Control and Prevention, July 27, 2022, https://www.cdc.gov/obesity/data/childhood.html.

4 *significant lifelong health consequences:* "Consequences of Obesity," Overweight and Obesity, Centers for Disease Control and Prevention, July 27, 2022, https://www.cdc.gov/obesity/data/childhood.html.

Chapter 5: The Dangers of Rewriting

1 *That seems to be a pretty strange line to draw:* "Childhood Obesity Facts," Overweight and Obesity, Centers for Disease Control and Prevention, July 27, 2022, https://www.cdc.gov/obesity/data/childhood.html.

PART TWO: FROM WHAT THEY'RE DOING TO WHAT YOU'RE DOING

1 *"social media makes it extraordinarily easy":* Greg Lukianoff and Jonathan Haidt, "The Coddling of the American Mind," *Atlantic,* August 11, 2015, https://www.theatlantic.com/magazine/archive/2015/09/the-coddling-of-the-american-mind/399356/.

2 *Instead, they want to engage in:* Jonathan Rauch, *Kindly Inquisitors: The New Attacks on Free Thought* (Chicago: University of Chicago Press, 2014), https://press.uchicago.edu/ucp/books/book/chicago/K/bo18140749.html.

Chapter 6: Deprogram Yourself, Because the Truth Is Out There

1 *A couple of professors:* Megan McArdle, "We Finally Know for Sure That Lies Spread Faster than the Truth. This Might Be Why," *Washington Post,* March 15, 2018, https://www.washingtonpost.com/opinions/we-finally-know-for-sure-that-lies-spread-faster-than-the-truth-this-might-be-why/2018/03/14/92ab1aae-27a6-11e8-bc72-077aa4dab9ef_story.html.

2 *I want you to read how they summarized:* Soroush Vosoughi, Deb Roy, and Sinan Aral, "The Spread of True and False News Online," *Science* 359, no. 6380 (March 9, 2018): 1146–51, https://doi.org/10.1126/science.aap9559.

Chapter 7: We're Doing Our Enemies' Work for Them

1 *Because it's working, on us, right now:* Paul Ratner, "39 Years Ago, a KGB Defector Chillingly Predicted Modern America," *Big Think* (blog), January 13, 2023, https://bigthink.com/the-present/yuri-bezmenov/.

2 *As Chase told me:* Conversation with Chase Hughes, April 20, 2023.

3 *The goal, according to both the guide and Bezmenov:* Ratner, "39 Years Ago, a KGB Defector Chillingly Predicted Modern America."

Chapter 8: Programmed by Algorithm (You're Angry, They Profit)

1 *In fact, none of us knew it:* Jeremy B. Merrill and William Oremus, "Five Points for Anger, One for a 'Like': How Facebook's Formula Fostered Rage and Misinformation," *Washington Post*, October 26, 2021, https://www .washingtonpost.com/technology/2021/10/26/facebook-angry-emoji-algo rithm/.

2 *That's right, the average American:* "The New Normal: Phone Use Is Up Nearly 4-Fold Since 2019, According to Tech Care Company Asurion," Asurion, April 22, 2022, https://www.asurion.com/connect/news/tech-usage/.

3 *When phones are silenced:* Mengqi Liao and S. Shyam Sundar, "Sound of Silence: Does Muting Notifications Reduce Phone Use?" *Computers in Human Behavior* 134 (September 1, 2022), https://doi.org/10.1016 /j.chb.2022.107338.

4 *And two-thirds of children spend:* Josh Howarth, "57+ Incredible Smartphone Addiction Statistics for 2023," Exploding Topics, February 2, 2023, https:// explodingtopics.com/blog/smartphone-addiction-stats.

5 *In 2023, America's surgeon general:* Teddy Amenabar, "What the Surgeon General's Advisory Says about Social Media for Kids," *Washington Post*, May 23, 2023, https://www.washingtonpost.com/wellness/2023/05/23/social-media -surgeon-general-youth-health-risk/.

6 *In one dramatic example, Target:* Kashmir Hill, "How Target Figured Out a Teen Girl Was Pregnant Before Her Father Did," *Forbes*, February 16, 2012, https://www.forbes.com/sites/kashmirhill/2012/02/16/how-target-figured -out-a-teen-girl-was-pregnant-before-her-father-did/.

Chapter 9: Censored by the Algorithm

1 *The way to know:* Natan Sharansky and Ron Dermer, *The Case for Democracy: The Power of Freedom to Overcome Tyranny and Terror* (New York: Public-Affairs, 2006), 40–41.

Chapter 10: Avoid Logical Fallacies: Presentism, Confirmation Bias, and Positive Bias

1 *It was about removing a statue of Thomas Jefferson:* "Canceling Thomas Jefferson," *National Review*, October 21, 2021, https://www.nationalreview.com /2021/10/canceling-thomas-jefferson/.

2 *Now say you have a Blue Lives Matter:* "Officer Deaths by Year," National Law Enforcement Officers Memorial Fund, March 24, 2023, https://nleomf.org /memorial/facts-figures/officer-fatality-data/officer-deaths-by-year/.

3 *If you're in the "all cops are bad" school of thought:* "Number of Full-Time Law Enforcement Officers in the United States from 2004 to 2021," Statista, 2023, https://www.statista.com/statistics/191694/number-of-law-enforce ment-officers-in-the-us/; Rich Morin and Andrew Mercer, "A Closer Look at Police Officers Who Have Fired Their Weapon on Duty," Pew Research Center, February 8, 2017, https://www.pewresearch.org/short-reads/2017/02/08 /a-closer-look-at-police-officers-who-have-fired-their-weapon-on-duty/.

4 *Or that you, the taxpayer:* Keith L. Alexander, Steven Rich, and Hannah Thacker, "The Hidden Billion-Dollar Cost of Repeated Police Misconduct," *Washington Post*, March 9, 2022, https://www.washingtonpost.com/investigations/inter active/2022/police-misconduct-repeated-settlements/; Morin and Mercer, "A Closer Look at Police Officers Who Have Fired Their Weapon on Duty."

5 *In his autobiography, Michael Eisner:* Malcolm Gladwell, "Was Jack Welch the Greatest C.E.O. of His Day—or the Worst?" *New Yorker*, October 31, 2022, https://www.newyorker.com/magazine/2022/11/07/was-jack-welch-the -greatest-ceo-of-his-day-or-the-worst.

6 *Listen to Burt Ross:* "Investors' Stories: How Bernard Madoff Stole Their Wealth and Their Dreams," *Frontline*, PBS, May 12, 2009, https://www.pbs .org/wgbh/pages/frontline/madoff/investors/.

Chapter 11: Are You Open to Changing Your Mind?

1 *In the 1970s, researchers surveyed:* Nikolas Westerhoff, "The 'Big Five' Person-ality Traits," *Scientific American*, December 17, 2008, https://www.scientific american.com/article/the-big-five/.

Chapter 12: The Dangerous Temptation of Victimhood

1 *I want you to take a moment and pull out a pencil:* Scott Barry Kaufman, "Unraveling the Mindset of Victimhood," *Scientific American*, June 29, 2020, https://www.scientificamerican.com/article/unraveling-the-mindset -of-victimhood/.

2 *In the late 1980s, Dr. Robert Kleck:* Sandra Blakeslee, "How You See Yourself: Potential for Big Problems," *New York Times*, February 7, 1991, https://www .nytimes.com/1991/02/07/news/how-you-see-yourself-potential-for-big -problems.html.

3 *To me, that's why Critical Race Theory:* "What Is Critical Race Theory and Why Is It in the News So Much?" ADL Education, November 15, 2021, https://www.adl.org/resources/tools-and-strategies/what-critical-race-theory -and-why-it-news-so-much.

4 *A culture of victimization led to the creation:* Nicole Chavez and Justin Gam- ble, "San Francisco Reparations Committee Proposes a $5 million Payment to Each Black Resident," CNN, January 19, 2023, https://www.cnn.com /2023/01/19/us/san-francisco-reparations-proposal-reaj/index.html.

5 *Dr. Kimmel had a defining moment:* "Dr. James Kimmel's Defining Moment," Phil in the Blanks, YouTube, 2022, https://www.youtube.com /watch?v=mQLuPcljpeg.

Chapter 13: Sociograms and Collective Personality

1 *I'm guessing the people of Portland:* Mike Baker, "An 'Army' of Volunteer Sleuths Is Out Hunting for Your Stolen Car," *New York Times*, October 29, 2022, https://www.nytimes.com/2022/10/29/us/portland-car-thefts-crime .html.

PART THREE: FAMILY, FAITH, AND COMMUNITY

Chapter 14: The Family Is Under Attack

1 *And here's the debris:* "Child Well-Being in Single-Parent Families," Annie E. Casey Foundation, August 1, 2022, https://www.aecf.org/blog/child-well -being-in-single-parent-families.

2 *As one example, single parents:* Natalie Stokes et al., "The Effect of the Lone Parent Household on Cardiovascular Health (National Health and Nutri- tion Examination Survey, 2015–2016)," *American Heart Journal Plus: Car-*

diology Research and Practice 3, no. 100015 (March 1, 2021), https://doi.org /10.1016/j.ahjo.2021.100015.

3   *Fewer children overall slows the economy:* "The Long-Term Decline in Fertility—and What It Means for State Budgets," Pew Charitable Trusts, December 5, 2022, https://pew.org/3VfmME1.

4   *Let's look a little deeper:* Gretchen Livingston, "The Changing Profile of Unmarried Parents," Pew Research Center, April 25, 2018, https://www .pewresearch.org/social-trends/2018/04/25/the-changing-profile-of-unmarried -parents/.

5   *In the 1960s, 73 percent:* "Parenting in America," Pew Research Center, December 17, 2015, https://www.pewresearch.org/social-trends/2015/12/17 /1-the-american-family-today/.

6   *The share of children living in a two-parent household:* Wendy Wang, "The Majority of U.S. Children Still Live in Two-Parent Families," Institute for Family Studies, October 4, 2018, https://ifstudies.org/blog/the-majority-of -us-children-still-live-in-two-parent-families.

7   *Here's another statistic:* "Parenting in America."

8   *A child with a biological mother:* Patrick Fagan, "Marriage: The Safest Place for Women and Children," Heritage Foundation, April 10, 2002, https:// www.heritage.org/welfare/report/marriage-the-safest-place-women-and-chil dren.

9   *And fatal assaults of young children by stepfathers:* Martin Daly and Margo Wilson, "The 'Cinderella Effect': Elevated Mistreatment of Stepchildren in Comparison to Those Living with Genetic Parents," Center for Evolutionary Psychology, University of California, Santa Barbara, n.d., https://live-center -for-evolutionary-psychology.pantheonsite.io/wp-content/uploads/2023/05 /cinderella-effect-facts.pdf.

10 *In fact, abuse or even murder:* Kristina Block and Jacob Kaplan, "Testing the Cinderella Effect: Measuring Victim Injury in Child Abuse Cases," *Journal of Criminal Justice* 82, no. 101987 (September 1, 2022), https://doi.org/10 .1016/j.jcrimjus.2022.101987.

11 *children living with their married biological parents:* Diana Zuckerman and Sarah Pedersen, "Child Abuse and Father Figures: Which Kind of Families Are Safest to Grow Up In?" National Center for Health Research, May 4, 2010, https://www.center4research.org/child-abuse-father-figures-kind-families -safest-grow/.

12 *Adult children of divorce:* "The Impact of Divorce on Children," Life-Giving Wounds, n.d., https://www.lifegivingwounds.org/research.

13 *In reality, it's more like 25 percent:* Renée Peltz Dennison, "Do Half of All Marriages Really End in Divorce?" *Psychology Today*, April 24, 2017, https://

www.psychologytoday.com/us/blog/heart-the-matter/201704/do-half-all
-marriages-really-end-in-divorce.

14 *Still, that's a lot, and this is a concern:* Felicitas Auersperg et al., "Long-Term
Effects of Parental Divorce on Mental Health: A Meta-Analysis," *Journal
of Psychiatric Research* 119 (December 1, 2019): 107–15, https://doi.org
/10.1016/j.jpsychires.2019.09.011; Kammi K. Schmeer, "Family Structure
and Obesity in Early Childhood," *Social Science Research* 41, no. 4 (July 1,
2012): 820–32, https://doi.org/10.1016/j.ssresearch.2012.01.007.

15 *Children of divorced or separated parents:* Brian D'Onofrio and Robert Emery,
"Parental Divorce or Separation and Children's Mental Health," *World Psychiatry* 18, no. 1 (February 2019): 100–101, https://doi.org/10.1002/wps
.20590.

16 *People need to get out of those marriages:* Jennie E. Brand et al., "Parental
Divorce Is Not Uniformly Disruptive to Children's Educational Attainment,"
Proceedings of the National Academy of Sciences 116, no. 15 (April 9, 2019):
7266–71, https://doi.org/10.1073/pnas.1813049116.

17 *Today, marriage is more about:* Andrew J. Cherlin, "The Deinstitutionalization
of American Marriage," *Journal of Marriage and Family* 66, no. 4 (2004):
848–61, https://doi.org/10.1111/j.0022-2445.2004.00058.x.

18 *Another reason sociologists:* "The Demise of the Happy Two-Parent Home,"
Social Capital Project, July 2020, https://www.jec.senate.gov/public/_cache
/files/84d5b05b-1a58-4b3f-8c8d-2f94cfe4bb59/3-20-the-demise-of-the
-happy-two-parent-home.pdf.

19 *One of the theories:* "The Demise of the Happy Two-Parent Home."

20 *The data clearly show:* W. Bradford Wilcox and Nicholas H. Wolfinger, "Men
and Marriage: Debunking the Ball and Chain Myth," Institute for Family
Studies, n.d., https://ifstudies.org/ifs-admin/resources/men-and-marriage
-research-brief.pdf.

Chapter 15: What Are You Modeling?

1 *Another trend:* Lauren J. Felt and Michael B. Robb, "Technology Addiction:
Concern, Controversy, and Finding Balance," Executive Summary, Common
Sense Media, May 2016, https://www.commonsensemedia.org/sites/default
/files/research/report/2016_csm_technology_addiction_executive_summary
.pdf; "Social Media Fact Sheet," Pew Research Center, April 7, 2021, https://
www.pewresearch.org/internet/fact-sheet/social-media/.

2 *Just as an example:* Robert A. Pollak, "An Intergenerational Model of Domestic Violence," *Journal of Population Economics* 17, no. 2 (June 1, 2004):
311–29, https://doi.org/10.1007/s00148-003-0177-7.

Chapter 16: The Dangerous Erosion of Faith

1 *our commitment to organized religion:* Jones, "U.S. Church Membership Falls Below Majority for First Time."

2 *Even as our population grows:* Jessica Grose, "Lots of Americans Are Losing Their Religion. Have You?" *New York Times*, April 19, 2023, https://www.nytimes.com/2023/04/19/opinion/religion-america.html; Isabella Kasselstrand, Phil Zuckerman, and Ryan T. Cragun, *Beyond Doubt: The Secularization of Society* (New York: New York University Press, 2023).

3 *According to a* Frontiers in Psychology *study:* Agnieszka Bożek, Paweł F. Nowak, and Mateusz Blukacz, "The Relationship Between Spirituality, Health-Related Behavior, and Psychological Well-Being," *Frontiers in Psychology* 11 (2020), https://www.frontiersin.org/articles/10.3389/fpsyg.2020.01997.

4 *Adults who attended religious services:* Patrick Fagan and Althea Nagai, "Happiness by Family Structure and Religious Practice," Mapping America, Marriage and Religion Institute, n.d., https://marri.us/wp-content/uploads/MA-49-51-165.pdf.

5 *And actively religious adults:* "Religion's Relationship to Happiness, Civic Engagement and Health Around the World," Pew Research Center, January 31, 2019, https://www.pewresearch.org/religion/2019/01/31/religions-relationship-to-happiness-civic-engagement-and-health-around-the-world/.

6 *In a divided society:* "17.3: Sociological Perspectives on Religion," in *Introduction to Sociology: Understanding and Changing the Social World* (University of Minnesota Libraries Publishing, 2016), https://open.lib.umn.edu/sociology/chapter/17-3-sociological-perspectives-on-religion/.

7 *teach people how to be good members of society:* "17.1: Sociological Perspectives on Religion," in *Introduction to Sociology*, https://pressbooks.howardcc.edu/soci101/.

8 Judges 17:6 (KJV).

9 Proverbs 12:15 (KJV).

10 *Homicide is rampant:* Joseph Chamie, "America's High Homicide Rate," N-IUSSP, February 6, 2023, https://www.niussp.org/health-and-mortality/americas-high-homicide-rate/.

11 Target has reported: "Target Wrestles with Pullback in Spending and Theft That May Cost It More than $1B This Year," NBC News, May 17, 2023, https://www.nbcnews.com/business/corporations/target-rising-costs-and-rising-theft-may-cost-1-billion-this-year-rcna84987; "Retailers Lost Up to $80 billion to Theft in 2022—Up by $13 billion in a Year," *Daily Mail*, September 27, 2023, https://www.dailymail.co.uk/yourmoney/article-12567059

/Retailers-lost-80-billion-shoplifting-13-billion-year.html?ito=email_share
_article-top.

12 *In New York:* Hurubie Meko, "A Tiny Number of Shoplifters Commit Thousands of New York City Thefts," *New York Times*, April 15, 2023, https://
www.nytimes.com/2023/04/15/nyregion/shoplifting-arrests-nyc.html.

13 Matthew 22:36–39.

Chapter 17: Science Is Under Attack

1 *Bud Light:* "Transgender Influencer Dylan Mulvaney Says Bud Light Didn't
Support Her during Backlash," AP News, June 30, 2023, https://apnews
.com/article/bud-light-transgender-dylan-mulvaney-442d6d4c3f41d
706586de8edd01ac13d.

2 *the case of transgender athletes:* Sophie Mann, "Majority of Americans Do
NOT Support Trans Athletes Competing against Women: Nearly 70% Say
Athletes Should Only Be Allowed to Compete on Sports Teams That Align
with Their Birth Gender, New Survey Shows," *Daily Mail*, June 12, 2023,
https://www.dailymail.co.uk/news/article-12186079/Majority-Americans
-NOT-support-trans-athletes-competing-against-women-new-survey-shows
.html.

3 *You don't need to hear many stories:* "Young Volleyball Star Who Was Injured
When Trans Player Spiked a Ball at Her Head Accuses Biden Administration
of 'Hypocrisy' after Karine Jean-Pierre Called Opposition to Transgender
Athletes in Girls' Sports 'Dangerous,'" *Daily Mail*, June 16, 2023, https://
www.dailymail.co.uk/news/article-12204921/High-school-volleyball-players
-speaks-transgender-athlete-issue.html.

4 *Even President Biden:* Sarah Mervosh, Remy Tumin, and Ava Sasani, "Biden
Plan Allows Limits on Trans Athletes' Participation in School Sports," *New
York Times*, April 6, 2023, https://www.nytimes.com/2023/04/06/us/trans
gender-athletes-title-ix-biden-adminstration.html.

5 *even with T blockers:* Doriane Lambelet Coleman and Wickliffe Shreve,
"Comparing Athletic Performances: The Best Elite Women to Boys and
Men," Duke Law, Center for Sports Law and Policy, n.d., https://law.duke
.edu/sports/sex-sport/comparative-athletic-performance/.

PART FOUR: THE TEN WORKING
PRINCIPLES FOR A HEALTHY SOCIETY

Principle #2: Focus on Solving Problems
Rather Than Winning Arguments

1 *Here's how they described it:* "Gates Foundation to Close Up 50 Years After Trustees' Deaths," *Education Week*, December 12, 2006, https://www .edweek.org/policy-politics/gates-foundation-to-close-up-50-years-after -trustees-deaths/2006/12.

2 *Right now in Texas:* James Lee, Pia Orrenius, and Ana Pranger, "Texas Birth-Rate Decline Complicates Economic Growth Prospects," Federal Reserve Bank of Dallas, October 12, 2021, https://www.dallasfed.org/research/eco nomics/2021/1012.

3 *This infuriated the police officers:* Mo Barnes, "Abusive Detroit Police Officers Mess with the Wrong Brothers," Rolling Out, September 15, 2014, https:// rollingout.com/2014/09/15/brothers-beat-abusive-detroit-thug-police/.

4 *A while back:* "'Fist Fight with Police' in Black and Blue: Race Relations in America," *Dr. Phil*, CBS, December 12, 2014, https://www.drphil.com /shows/2329/.

5 *In the decade between 2012 and 2022:* Keith L. Alexander, Steven Rich, and Hannah Thacker, "The Hidden Billion-Dollar Cost of Repeated Police Misconduct," *Washington Post*, March 9, 2022, https://www.washingtonpost.com /investigations/interactive/2022/police-misconduct-repeated-settlements/.

Principle #3: Don't Reward Bad Behavior or
Support Conduct You Do Not Value

1 *Harm reduction policies and approaches:* "What is Harm Reduction?" Harm Reduction International, n.d., https://hri.global/what-is-harm-reduction/.

2 *In 2022, the last year for which:* "Drug Overdose Death Rates," National Institute on Drug Abuse, June 30, 2023, https://nida.nih.gov/research-topics /trends-statistics/overdose-death-rates; Luke Andrews, "Drug Overdoses Killed Equivalent of Airliner Full of Americans Every DAY Last Year, New Figures Show," *Daily Mail*, May 19, 2023, https://www.dailymail.co.uk /news/article-11929519/Federal-judges-announce-refuse-hire-clerks-Stan ford-Law-School-woke-students.html?ito=email_share_article-top.

3 *As the biomedical ethicist Nicholas King:* Nicholas B. King, "Harm Reduction:

A Misnomer," *Health Care Analysis* 28, no. 4 (2020): 324–34, https://doi.org
/10.1007/s10728-020-00413-x.

4   *One study found that fewer than 7 percent:* Steven Bozza and Jeffrey Berger,
"Safe Injection Sites: A Moral Reflection," *Linacre Quarterly* 87, no. 1 (February 1, 2020): 85–93, https://doi.org/10.1177/0024363919861590.

5   *They don't focus on restoring:* Bozza and Berger.

Principle #4: Measure All Actions Based on Results, and All Thoughts Based on Rationality

1   *More than 40 percent:* Chloe Haderlie and Alyssa Clark, "Illiteracy Among
Adults in the United States," Ballard Brief, n.d., https://ballardbrief.byu.edu
/issue-briefs/illiteracy-among-adults-in-the-us.

2   *Early in 2023, the Illinois:* "Report Card Data Library," Illinois State Board of
Education, January 19, 2023, https://www.isbe.net.

3   *Wirepoints says that its mission:* "About Us," Wirepoints, October 19, 2019,
https://wirepoints.org/about-us-2/.

4   *In Baltimore, twenty-three schools:* Chris Papst, "23 Baltimore Schools Have
Zero Students Proficient in Math, per State Test Results," FOX45 News Baltimore, February 6, 2023, https://foxbaltimore.com/news/project-baltimore
/state-test-results-23-baltimore-schools-have-zero-students-proficient-in
-math-jovani-patterson-maryland-comprehensive-assessment-program
-maryland-governor-wes-moore.

5   *Richard Feynman:* Richard Feynman, "Seeking New Laws," Messenger Lectures on the Character of Physical Law, Cornell University, November 9,
1964, https://jamesclear.com/great-speeches/seeking-new-laws-by-richard
-feynman.

6   *His expertise was physics:* Richard Feynman, "Cargo-Cult Science Speech,"
commencement speech, California Institute of Technology, 1974, https://
goodonewilson.substack.com/embed.

7   *During World War II:* Peter M. Worsley, "50 Years Ago: Cargo Cults of Mela-
nesia," *Scientific American*, May 1, 2009, https://www.scientificamerican
.com/article/1959-cargo-cults-melanesia/.

8   *This is the highest level of teenage sadness:* Derek Thompson, "Why American
Teens Are So Sad," *Atlantic*, April 11, 2022, https://www.theatlantic.com
/newsletters/archive/2022/04/american-teens-sadness-depression-anxiety
/629524/.

9   *The total number of teenagers:* A. W. Geiger and Leslie Davis, "A Growing
Number of American Teenagers—Particularly Girls—Are Facing Depression," Pew Research Center, July 12, 2019, https://www.pewresearch.org

/short-reads/2019/07/12/a-growing-number-of-american-teenagers-particu larly-girls-are-facing-depression/.

10 *And that doesn't even begin to touch:* Claudia Goldin, "Understanding the Economic Impact of COVID-19 on Women," Working Paper, National Bureau of Economic Research, April 2022, https://doi.org/10.3386/w29974.

11 *a quarter of them wanted:* Gema Zamarro et al., "How the Pandemic Has Changed Teachers' Commitment to Remaining in the Classroom," Brookings Institution, September 8, 2021, https://www.brookings.edu/articles /how-the-pandemic-has-changed-teachers-commitment-to-remaining-in -the-classroom/.

12 *The problem was not with the teachers:* Bradley Marianno, "Teachers' Unions: Scapegoats or Bad-Faith Actors in COVID-19 School Reopening Decisions?" Brookings Institution, March 25, 2021, https://www.brookings.edu /articles/teachers-unions-scapegoats-or-bad-faith-actors-in-covid-19-school -reopening-decisions/.

13 *The models predict that the toll:* Dimitri A. Christakis, Wil Van Cleve, and Frederick J. Zimmerman, "Estimation of US Children's Educational Attainment and Years of Life Lost Associated with Primary School Closures During the Coronavirus Disease 2019 Pandemic," *Journal of the American Medical Association* 3, no. 11 (November 2, 2020), https://doi.org/10.1001/jamanet workopen.2020.28786.

14 *Sadly, some surveys:* Anjali Sundaram, "Yelp Data Shows 60% of Business Closures Due to the Coronavirus Pandemic Are Now Permanent," CNBC, September 16, 2020, https://www.cnbc.com/2020/09/16/yelp-data-shows -60percent-of-business-closures-due-to-the-coronavirus-pandemic-are-now -permanent.html.

15 *So even after a vaccine was available:* Anousha Sakoui, "What Is a COVID-19 Compliance Supervisor? What to Know about Hollywood's Newest Job," *Los Angeles Times*, October 27, 2020, https://www.latimes.com/entertainment -arts/business/story/2020-10-27/covid-compliance-supervisors-hollywood -pandemic.

Principle #6: Do Not Stay Silent Just So Others Can Remain Comfortable

1 *Nearly two-thirds of Americans:* Emily Ekins, "Poll: 62% of Americans Say They Have Political Views They're Afraid to Share," Cato Institute, July 22, 2020, https://www.cato.org/survey-reports/poll-62-americans-say -they-have-political-views-theyre-afraid-share.

2 *More than half of college students:* "College Free Speech Rankings: What's the

Climate for Free Speech on America's College Campuses?" College Pulse, FIRE, and RealClear Education, 2021, https://f.hubspotusercontent00.net /hubfs/5666503/2021_Campus%20Free%20Speech%20Report.pdf.

3 *However, there is substantial:* Ekins, "Poll."

4 *This leads people:* Michael Chan, "Reluctance to Talk About Politics in Face-to-Face and Facebook Settings: Examining the Impact of Fear of Isolation, Willingness to Self-Censor, and Peer Network Characteristics," *Mass Communication and Society* 21, no. 1 (January 2, 2018): 1–23, https://doi.org /10.1080/15205436.2017.1358819.

5 *One study found that when groups:* Alice E. Marwick, "Morally Motivated Networked Harassment as Normative Reinforcement," *Social Media + Society* 7, no. 2 (April 2021): 205630512110213, https://doi.org/10.1177 /20563051211021378.

6 *But I found one study:* Femke Geusens, Gaëlle Ouvrein, and Soetkin Remen, "#Cancelled: A Qualitative Content Analysis of Cancel Culture in the YouTube Beauty Community," *Social Science Journal*, February 15, 2023, 1–17, https://doi.org/10.1080/03623319.2023.2175150.

7 *In 1997, Michigan State University:* Julie Mack, "Nassar Victim Describes Telling MSU Coach in 1997 about Abuse," MLive, January 19, 2018, https://www.mlive.com/news/2018/01/nassar_victim_describes_tellin.html.

8 *And whoever does the procedure:* Roni Caryn Rabin, "Pelvic Massage Can Be Legitimate, but Not in Larry Nassar's Hands," *New York Times*, January 31, 2018, https://www.nytimes.com/2018/01/31/well/live/pelvic-massage-can -be-legitimate-but-not-in-larry-nassars-hands.html.

9 *Dr. James Heaps:* Emily Olson, "Court Finds Former UCLA Gynecologist Guilty of Sexually Abusing Patients," NPR, October 21, 2022, https://www .npr.org/2022/10/21/1130449690/ucla-gynecologist-guilty-sexual-abuse -metoo.

10 *The impact statements:* Kelly Wynne, "Why Larry Nassar Sentencing Judge Rosemarie Aquilina Let Victim Statements Last for Days," *Newsweek*, May 3, 2019, https://www.newsweek.com/larry-nassar-sentencing-judge-rosemarie -aquilina-talks-victim-statements-1412869.

11 *She decided her courtroom:* Wynne.

Principle #7: Actively Live and Support a Meritocracy

1 *I'm sure you've heard:* Phil Gramm and John Early, "Incredible Shrinking Income Inequality," *Wall Street Journal*, March 23, 2021, https://www.wsj .com/articles/incredible-shrinking-income-inequality-11616517284.

2 *So, your government makes:* Gramm and Early.

3 *In chapter 2, I mentioned that when Michael Eisner:* Gladwell, "Was Jack Welch the Greatest C.E.O. of His Day—or the Worst?"

4 *Lowering Standards in the Classroom:* Nicholas Giordano, "The Biggest Scandal in Higher Education Is Lowering the Bar," Fox News, October 7, 2022, https://www.foxnews.com/opinion/biggest-scandal-higher-education-lowering-bar.

5 *Meet Maitland Jones Jr.:* Nour Che, "8 of the Coolest Professors at NYU," *OneClass* (blog), September 18, 2017, https://oneclass.com/blog/new-york-university/9997-8-of-the-coolest-professors-at-nyu.en.html.

6 *But Dr. Jones started to notice:* Stephanie Saul, "At N.Y.U., Students Were Failing Organic Chemistry. Who Was to Blame?" *New York Times*, October 3, 2022, https://www.nytimes.com/2022/10/03/us/nyu-organic-chemistry-petition.html.

7 *A former chairman:* Saul.

8 *After all this, several students told:* Faye Flam, "An NYU Professor Got Fired. Then Everyone Missed the Point," *Washington Post*, October 12, 2022, https://www.washingtonpost.com/business/an-nyu-professor-got-fired-then-everyone-missed-the-point/2022/10/12/5913084e-4a36-11ed-8153-96ee97b218d2_story.html.

9 *Companies institute these programs:* Janice Gassam Asare, "4 Ways the Supreme Court's Affirmative Action Decision Could Impact Workplace DEI," *Forbes*, June 29, 2023, https://www.forbes.com/sites/janicegassam/2023/06/29/4-ways-the-supreme-courts-affirmative-action-decision-could-impact-workplace-dei/.

10 *In 2022, New York City:* Katie Honan, "City Makes Swim Test Easier to Mind Mini Pools," The City, July 6, 2023, https://www.thecity.nyc/2022/7/8/23200593/nyc-makes-swim-test-easier-to-mind-mini-pools.

11 *According to the Associated Press:* Adrian Sainz, Jim Mustian, and Bernard Condon, "Amid Soaring Crime, Memphis Cops Lowered the Bar for Hiring," AP News, February 7, 2023, https://apnews.com/article/law-enforcement-tyre-nichols-memphis-crime-93033874b99a4893c6c996fd56676795.

12 *Cancel culture went crazy:* Tyler Jenke, "Sia Criticised for Autism Representation in Upcoming Film, 'Music,'" *Rolling Stone Australia* (blog), November 20, 2020, https://au.rollingstone.com/music/music-news/sia-criticised-autism-representation-music-19614/.

13 *Amid the controversy:* Alexander Pan, "Sia Defends Casting Neurotypical Maddie Ziegler as Autistic Lead in Music," *The Brag* (blog), December 17, 2020, https://thebrag.com/sia-defends-neurotypical-maddie-ziegler-music-film/.

14 *Helen Mirren took a lot of heat:* Samantha Bergeson, "Helen Mirren Breaks

Silence About 'Unfairness' Surrounding Golda Meir Casting Controversy," IndieWire, February 7, 2022, https://www.indiewire.com/features /general/helen-mirren-golda-meir-casting-controversy-jewish-unfairness -1234697048/.

Principle #8: Identify and Build
Your Consequential Knowledge

1 *But it's now estimated:* Sebastien Bell, "Autonomous Trucks Could Replace 90% of Humans on Long-Haul Routes," Carscoops, March 21, 2022, https://www.carscoops.com/2022/03/autonomous-trucks-could-replace -90-of-humans-on-long-haul-routes/.

2 *And then in the future:* David Edwards, "Automation Isn't About to Make Truckers Obsolete," *Robotics & Automation News*, February 23, 2022, https:// roboticsandautomationnews.com/2022/02/23/automation-isnt-about-to -make-truckers-obsolete/49489/.

3 *Roughly 3 million Americans:* "Number of Contact Center Employees in the United States from 2014 to 2022," Statista, March 2023, https://www .statista.com/statistics/881114/contact-center-employees-united-states/.

4 *In fact, it's estimated that automation:* Jack Flynn, "35+ Alarming Automation & Job Loss Statistics [2023]: Are Robots, Machines, and AI Coming For Your Job?" *Zippia* (blog), June 8, 2023, https://www.zippia.com/advice /automation-and-job-loss-statistics/.

5 *In 1900, roughly 40 percent:* Jayson Lusk, "The Evolution of American Agriculture," June 27, 2016, http://jaysonlusk.com/blog/2016/6/26/the-evolution -of-american-agriculture.

6 *Now, as I'm writing this book:* Carlos Granda, "Higher Fees for Borrowers with Good Credit? Inside Biden's New Rules on Mortgage Fees," ABC7 Los Angeles, April 28, 2023, https://abc7.com/joe-biden-mortgage-fees-policy -homeowners-first-time-buyer/13190960/.

7 *In the early 1960s:* Dennis Hevesi, "Arch West, Who Helped Create Doritos Corn Chips, Is Dead at 97," *New York Times*, September 28, 2011, https:// www.nytimes.com/2011/09/28/business/arch-west-who-helped-create-doritos -corn-chips-is-dead-at-97.html.

8 *Taking a risk, inventing a new product:* Katie Daubs, "No Cheesy Farewell for Doritos Creator," *Toronto Star*, September 27, 2011, https://www.thestar.com /news/world/2011/09/27/no_cheesy_farewell_for_doritos_creator.html.

9 *When Arch died in 2011:* Marice Richter, "Doritos Founder to Be Buried with Iconic Snack Chips," Reuters, September 28, 2011, https://www.reuters.com /article/us-doritos-burial-idUSTRE78R22V20110928.

10 *In the late 1960s and early 1970s:* Janine Zacharia, "The Bing 'Marshmallow Studies': 50 Years of Continuing Research," Stanford University Bing Nursery School, September 24, 2015, https://bingschool.stanford.edu/news/bing-marshmallow-studies-50-years-continuing-research.

11 *If they waited for him:* David Brooks, "Marshmallows and Public Policy," *New York Times*, May 7, 2006, https://www.nytimes.com/2006/05/07/opinion/07brooks.html.

Principle #9: Work Hard to Understand the Way Others See Things

1 *He and I still share:* Molly Ball, "The Agony of Frank Luntz," *Atlantic*, January 6, 2014, https://www.theatlantic.com/politics/archive/2014/01/the-agony-of-frank-luntz/282766/.

2 *So, in recent years:* Ariel Zilber, "Tucker Carlson Claims Powerful GOP Pollster Frank Luntz Is Secret LIBERAL and Blasts Him for Pushing Pro-Immigration Policies," *Daily Mail*, April 30, 2021, https://www.dailymail.co.uk/news/article-9531883/Tucker-Carlson-claims-powerful-GOP-pollster-Frank-Luntz-secret-LIBERAL.html.

3 *And I'm worried because even tragedies:* Toluse Olorunnipa, Justine McDaniel, and Ian Duncan, "How a Small-Town Train Derailment Erupted into a Culture Battle," *Washington Post*, February 25, 2023, https://www.washingtonpost.com/politics/2023/02/25/derailment-east-palestine-culture-wars/.

Principle #10: Treat Yourself and Others with Dignity and Respect

1 *So the FAA put in place:* Terry Castleman, "Unruly Airplane Passengers Disrupting More Flights, Despite FAA's Zero-Tolerance Policy," *Los Angeles Times*, June 6, 2023, https://www.latimes.com/world-nation/story/2023-06-06/unruly-passenger-incidents-on-airplanes-up-47-last-year-worldwide.

Conclusion: Step onto the Number Line

1 *It's part of why seven out of every ten:* "NBC News Survey," Hart Research Associates and Public Opinion Strategies, January 2023, https://s3.documentcloud.org/documents/23589424/230032-nbc-january-2023-poll-v2-129-release.pdf.